PEDIATRICS, CHILD AND ADOLESCENT HEALTH

BUILDING CHILDREN AND YOUTH FOR THE FUTURE

SOME INTERNATIONAL ASPECTS

PEDIATRICS, CHILD AND ADOLESCENT HEALTH

JOAV MERRICK - SERIES EDITOR

NATIONAL INSTITUTE OF CHILD HEALTH AND HUMAN DEVELOPMENT, MINISTRY OF SOCIAL AFFAIRS, JERUSALEM

Building Children and Youth for the Future: Some International Aspects
Joav Merrick, Ariel Tenenbaum Hatim A Omar (Editors)
2021. ISBN: 978-1-53618-806-6 (Hardcover)
2021. ISBN: 978-1-53619-017-5 (e-book)

Tropical Pediatrics: a Public Health Concern of International Proportions, 3rd Edition
Richard R Roach, Donald E Greydanus, Dilip R Patel, and Joav Merrick (Editors)
2021. ISBN: 978-1-53618-604-8 (Hardcover)
2021. ISBN: 978-1-53618-928-5 (e-book)

Childhood and Adolescence: Perspectives of Pain
Donald E Greydanus and Joav Merrick (Editors)
2020: ISBN 978-1-53618-416-7 (Hardcover)

Adolescence: International Aspects of Interpersonal and Self-Directed Violence
Supa Pengpid, Karl Peltzer and Joav Merrick (Editors)
2020. ISBN: 978-1-53618-066-4 (Softcover)
2020. ISBN: 978-1-53618-067-1 (e-book)

School Health in Asia and Africa
Supa Pengpid, Karl Peltzer and Joav Merrick (Editors)
2020. ISBN: 978-1-53617-868-5 (Hardcover)
2020. ISBN: 978-1-53617-869-2 (e-book)

Chronic Disease and Disability: The Pediatric Liver
Donald E Greydanus, Ransome Eke, Orhan Atay and Joav Merrick (Editors)
2020. ISBN: 978-1-53617-750-3 (Hardcover)
2020. ISBN: 978-1-53617-751-0 (e-book)

Chronic Disease and Disability: The Pediatric Heart, Second Edition
Donald E Greydanus, Premchand Anne, John D. Rowlett and Joav Merrick (Editors)
2020. ISBN: 978-1-53617-656-8 (Hardcover)
2020. ISBN: 978-1-53617-657-5 (e-book)

Adolescence: Behavioural Risk Factors of Non-Communicable Diseases
Supa Pengpid, Karl Peltzer and Joav Merrick (Editors)
2020. ISBN: 978-1-53617-704-6 (Hardcover)
2020. ISBN: 978-1-53617-705-3 (e-book)

Adolescence in Curaçao
Soraya Verstraeten, Supa Pengpid, Karl Peltzer and Joav Merrick (Editors)
2020. ISBN: 978-1-53617-522-6 (Softcover)
2020. ISBN: 978-1-53617-523-3 (e-book)

Building Youth for the Future: Suicide Prevention Aspects
Hatim A. Omar and Joav Merrick (Editors)
2019. ISBN: 978-1-53615-799-4 (Hardcover)
2019. ISBN: 978-1-53616-565-4 (e-book)

Vaccine: Measles and Rubella Vaccination Experience in Zambia
Mazyanga L. Mazaba-Liwewe, Seter Siziya and Joav Merrick (Editors)
2019. ISBN: 978-1-53615-799-4 (Hardcover)
2019. ISBN: 978-1-53615-800-7 (e-book)

The Boko Haram Terror: Adversary to the Wellbeing of Nigerian Kids
Miracle A. Adesina, Kehinde K. Kanmodi and Joav Merrick (Editors)
2019. ISBN: 978-1-53615-443-6 (Softcover)
2019. ISBN: 978-1-53615-444-3 (e-book)

Chronic Disease and Disability: Pediatric Obesity Perspectives
Marisha Agana, Donald E. Greydanus, Manmohan K. Kamboj and Joav Merrick (Editors)
2019. ISBN: 978-1-53615-240-1 (Hardcover)
2019. ISBN: 978-1-53615-241-8 (e-book)

Substance Use Disorders in Adolescents and Young Adults: A Manual for Pediatric and Primary Care Clinicians. Second Edition
Donald E. Greydanus, Gabriel Kaplan, Dilip R. Patel and Joav Merrick (Editors)
2019. ISBN: 978-1-53615-359-0 (Hardcover)
2019. ISBN: 978-1-53615-360-6 (e-book)

Building Youth for the Future: A Path towards Suicide Prevention
Hatim A. Omar and Joav Merrick (Editors)
2018. ISBN: 978-1-53613-768-2 (Hardcover)
2018. ISBN: 978-1-53613-769-9 (e-book)

Soft Skills and Aspirations in Chinese Children and Youth
Daniel T.L. Shek, Janet TY Leung and Joav Merrick (Editors)
2018. ISBN: 978-1-53614-092-7 (Hardcover)
2018. ISBN: 978-1-53614-093-4 (e-book)

Childhood and Adolescence: Tribute to Emanuel Chigier, 1928-2017
Joav Merrick (Editor)
2018. ISBN: 978-1-53613-574-9 (Hardcover)
2018. ISBN: 978-1-53613-574-9 (e-book)

Child Health and Human Development Yearbook 2017
Joav Merrick (Editor)
2018. ISBN: 978-1-53613-628-9 (Hardcover)
2018. ISBN: 978-1-53613-629-6 (e-book)

Child and Adolescent Health Yearbook 2017
Joav Merrick (Editor)
2018. ISBN: 978-1-53613-594-7 (Hardcover)
2018. ISBN: 978-1-53613-595-4 (e-book)

Chronic Disease and Disability: The Pediatric Gastrointestinal Tract
Donald E Greydanus, Orhan Atay, and Joav Merrick (Editors)
2018. ISBN: 978-1-53612-948-9 (Hardcover)
2018. ISBN: 978-1-53612-949-6 (e-book)

Multiple Sclerosis in Children and Adolescents
Hatim Omar and Joshua Chalkley (Editors)
2018. ISBN: 978-1-53612-979-3 (Hardcover)
2018. ISBN: 978-1-53612-980-9 (e-book)

Childhood and Adolescence: Tribute to Emanuel Chigier, 1928-2017
Joav Merrick (Editor)
2018. ISBN: 978-1-53613-574-9 (Softcover)
2018. ISBN: 978-1-53613-575-6 (e-book)

Chronic Disease and Disability: The Pediatric Lung
Donald E Greydanus, Myrtha M Gregoire-Bottex, Kevin W Cates and Joav Merrick (Editors)
2018. ISBN: 978-1-53613-577-0 (Hardcover)
2018. ISBN: 978-1-53613-578-7 (e-book)

Bicycles: Helmet Use of Adolescents at Independent Schools
Ronald Chow, Michael Borean, Drew Hollenberg, Jaclyn Viehweger, Tharani Anpalagan and Anna Rzepka (Editors)
2017. ISBN: 978-1-53612-458-3 (Hardcover)
2017. ISBN: 978-1-53612-459-0 (e-book)

Positive Youth Development: Long Term Effects in a Chinese Program
Daniel TL Shek, Cecilia MS Ma, Janet TY Leung and Joav Merrick (Editors)
2017. ISBN: 978-1-53612-539-9 (Hardcover)
2017. ISBN: 978-1-53612-540-5 (e-book)

Adolescence: Bicycle and Helmet Use of Adolescents and Young Adults
Ronald Chow and Joav Merrick (Editors)
2017. ISBN: 978-1-53612-039-4 (Hardcover)
2017. ISBN: 978-1-53612-060-8 (e-book)

Suicide: A Global View on Suicidal Ideation among Adolescents
Mazyanga L. Mazaba, Seter Siziya and Joav Merrick (Editors)
2017. ISBN: 978-1-53611-788-2 (Hardcover)
2017. ISBN: 978-1-53611-799-8 (e-book)

Children and Youth: Post-Traumatic Stress Disorder and Motor Vehicle Crashes
Donald E. Greydanus, Roger W. Apple, Kathryn White, and Joav Merrick (Editors)
2017. ISBN: 978-1-53611-102-6 (Hardcover)
2017. ISBN: 978-1-53611-255-9 (e-book)

Child and Adolescent Health Yearbook 2016
Joav Merrick (Editor)
2017. ISBN: 978-1-53610-948-1 (Hardcover)
2017. ISBN: 978-1-53610-957-3 (e-book)

Child Health and Human Development Yearbook 2016
Joav Merrick (Editor)
2017. ISBN: 978-1-53610-946-7 (Hardcover)
2017. ISBN: 978-1-53610-958-0 (e-book)

Chronic Disease and Disability: The Pediatric Kidney
Donald E Greydanus, Vimal Master Sankar Raj, and Joav Merrick (Editors)
2016. ISBN: 978-1-63483-793-4 (Hardcover)
2015. ISBN: 978-1-63483-809-2 (e-book)

Child and Adolescent Health Yearbook 2015
Joav Merrick (Editor)
2016. ISBN: 978-1-63484-512-0 (Hardcover)
2016. ISBN: 978-1-63484-543-4 (e-book)

Child Health and Human Development Yearbook 2015
Joav Merrick (Editor)
2016. ISBN: 978-1-63484-513-7 (Hardcover)
2016. ISBN: 978-1-63484-544-1 (e-book)

Pain Management Yearbook 2015
Joav Merrick (Editor)
2016. ISBN: 978-1-63484-515-1 (Hardcover)
2016. ISBN: 978-1-63484-545-8 (e-book)

Children and Childhood: Some International Aspects
Joav Merrick (Editor)
2016. ISBN: 978-1-63484-587-8 (Hardcover)
2016. ISBN: 978-1-63484-594-6 (e-book)

Children and Adolescents: Future Challenges
Daniel TL Shek, Tak Yan Lee, and Joav Merrick (Editors)
2016. ISBN: 978-1-63484-616-5 (Hardcover)
2016. ISBN: 978-1-63484-627-1 (e-book)

Adolescence: Positive Youth Development Programs in Chinese Communities
Daniel TL Shek, Florence KY Wu, Janet TY Leung, and Joav Merrick (Editors)
2016. ISBN: 978-1-63484-044-6 (Hardcover)
2016. ISBN: 978-1-63484-677-6 (e-book)

Growing Up in the Middle East: The Daily Lives and Well-Being of Israeli and Palestinian Youth
Yossi Harel-Fisch, Ziad Abdeen and Miriam Navot
2016. ISBN: 978-1-63484-746-9 (Hardcover)
2016. ISBN: 978-1-63484-765-0 (e-book)

Sexuality: Some International Aspects
Joav Merrick and Donald E Greydanus (Editors)
2016. ISBN: 978-1-63484-707-0 (Hardcover)
2016. ISBN: 978-1-63484-719-3 (e-book)

Chronic Disease and Disability: The Pediatric Heart
Donald E Greydanus, Devika Malhotra and Joav Merrick (Editors)
2016. ISBN: 978-1-63484-828-2 (Hardcover)
2016. ISBN: 978-1-63484-842-8 (e-book)

Diabetes Mellitus: Childhood and Adolescence
Manmohan K Kamboj, Donald E Greydanus and Joav Merrick (Editors)
2016. ISBN: 978-1-53610-095-2 (Hardcover)
2016. ISBN: 978-1-53610-104-1 (e-book)

Chronic Disease and Disability: Abuse and Neglect in Childhood and Adolescence
Donald E Greydanus, Vincent J Palusci and Joav Merrick (Editors)
2016. ISBN: 978-1-53610-129-4 (Hardcover)
2016. ISBN: 978-1-53610-142-3 (e-book)

Clinical Aspects of Psychopharmacology in Childhood and Adolescence, Second Edition
Donald E Greydanus, Joseph L Calles, Jr, Dilip R Patel, Ahsan Nazeer and Joav Merrick (Editors)
2016. ISBN: 978-1-53610-241-3 (Hardcover)
2016. ISBN: 978-1-53610-253-6 (e-book)

Chronic Disease and Disability: The Pediatric Pancreas
Donald E Greydanus, Manmohan K Kamboj and Joav Merrick (Editors)
2016. ISBN: 978-1-53610-055-6 (Hardcover)
2016. ISBN: 978-1-53610-065-5 (e-book)

A Pediatric Resident Pocket Guide: Making the Most of Morning Reports
Arthur N Feinberg
2015. ISBN: 978-1-63482-141-4 (Softcover)
2015. ISBN: 978-1-63482-186-5 (e-book)

Child and Adolescent Health Yearbook 2014
Joav Merrick (Editor)
2015. ISBN: 978-1-63482-162-9 (Hardcover)
2015. ISBN: 978-1-63482-206-0 (e-book)

Tropical Pediatrics: A Public Health Concern of International Proportions Second Edition
Richard R Roach, Donald E Greydanus, Dilip R Patel and Joav Merrick (Editors)
2015. ISBN: 978-1-63463-381-9 (Hardcover)
2015. ISBN: 978-1-63463-404-5 (c-book)

Child and Adolescent Health Issues (A Tribute to the Pediatrician Donald E Greydanus)
Joav Merrick (Editor)
2015. ISBN: 978-1-63463-574-5 (Hardcover)
2015. ISBN: 978-1-63463-576-9 (e-book)

Child Health and Human Development Yearbook 2014
Joav Merrick (Editor)
2015. ISBN: 978-1-63482-163-6 (Hardcover)
2015. ISBN: 978-1-63482-207-7 (e-book)

Behavioral Pediatrics, 4th Edition
Donald E Greydanus, Dilip R Patel, Helen D Pratt, Joseph L Calles Jr, Ahsan Nazeer and Joav Merrick (Editors)
2015. ISBN: 978-1-63483-027-0 (Hardcover)
2015. ISBN: 978-1-63483-052-2 (e-book)

Disability, Chronic Disease and Human Development
Joav Merrick
2015. ISBN: 978-1-63483-029-4 (Hardcover)
2015. ISBN: 978-1-63483-057-7 (e-book)

Caribbean Adolescents: Some Public Health Concerns
Cecilia Hegamin-Younge and Joav Merrick (Editors)
2015. ISBN: 978-1-63483-341-7 (Hardcover)
2015. ISBN: 978-1-63483-343-1 (e-book)

Adolescence and Health: Some International Perspectives
Joav Merrick (Editor)
2015. ISBN: 978-1-63483-791-0 (Hardcover)
2015. ISBN: 978-1-63483-808-5 (e-book)

Youth Suicide Prevention: Everybody's Business
Hatim A Omar (Editor)
2015. ISBN: 978-1-63483-786-6 (Softcover)
2015. ISBN: 978-1-63483-820-7 (e-book)

Human Developmental Research: Experience from Research in Hong Kong
Daniel TL Shek, Cecilia Ma, Yu Lu and Joav Merrick (Editors)
2014. ISBN: 978-1-62808-166-4 (Hardcover)
2013. ISBN: 978-1-62808-167-1 (e-book)

School, Adolescence and Health Issues
Joav Merrick, Ariel Tenenbaum and Hatim A Omar (Editors)
2014. ISBN: 978-1-62948-702-1 (Hardcover)
2014. ISBN: 978-1-62948-707-6 (e-book)

Adolescence and Sexuality: International Perspectives
Joav Merrick, Ariel Tenenbaum and Hatim A Omar (Editors)
2014. ISBN: 978-1-62948-711-3 (Hardcover)
2014. ISBN: 978-1-62948-724-3 (e-book)

Child and Adolescent Health Yearbook 2013
Joav Merrick (Editor)
2014. ISBN: 978-1-63117-658-6 (Hardcover)
2014. ISBN: 978-1-63117-668-5 (e-book)

Adoption: The Search for a New Parenthood
Gary Diamond and Eva Arbel
2014. ISBN: 978-1-63117-710-1 (Hardcover)
2014. ISBN: 978-1-63117-713-2 (e-book)

Adolescence: Places and Spaces
Myra F Taylor, Julie Ann Pooley and Joav Merrick (Editors)
2014. ISBN: 978-1-63117-847-4 (Hardcover)
2014. ISBN: 978-1-63117-850-4 (e-book)

Child Health and Human Development Yearbook 2013
Joav Merrick (Editor)
2014. ISBN: 978-1-63117-939-6 (Hardcover)
2013. ISBN: 978-1-63117-958-7 (e-book)

Born into this World: Health Issues
Donald E Greydanus, Arthur N Feinberg, and Joav Merrick (Editors)
2014. ISBN: 978-1-63321-667-9 (Hardcover)
2014. ISBN: 978-1-63321-669-3 (e-book)

Caring for the Newborn: A Comprehensive Guidc for the Clinician
Donald E Greydanus, Arthur N Feinberg and Joav Merrick (Editors)
2014. ISBN: 978-1-63321-760-7 (Hardcover)
2014. ISBN: 978-1-63321-781-2 (e-book)

Environment and Hope: Impoving Health, Reducing AIDS and Promoting Food Security in the World
Leslie Rubin and Joav Merrick (Editors)
2014. ISBN: 978-1-63321-772-0 (Hardcover)
2014. ISBN: 978-1-63321-782-9 (e-book)

Pain Management Yearbook 2013
Joav Merrick (Editor)
2014. ISBN: 978-1-63117-944-0 (Hardcover)
2014. ISBN: 978-1-63117-959-4 (e-book)

Pediatric and Adolescent Dermatology: Some Current Issues
Donald E Greydanus, Arthur N Feinberg and Joav Merrick (Editors)
2014. ISBN: 978-1-63321-853-6 (Hardcover)
2014. ISBN: 978-1-63321-863-5 (e-book)

Adolescence and Behavior Issues in a Chinese Context
Daniel TL Shek, Rachel CF Sun, and Joav Merrick (Editors)
2013. ISBN: 978-1-62618-614-9 (Hardcover)
2013. ISBN: 978-1-62618-692-7 (e-book)

Advances in Preterm Infant Research
Jing Sun, Nicholas Buys and Joav Merrick
2013. ISBN: 978-1-62618-696-5 (Hardcover)
2013. ISBN: 978-1-62618-775-7 (e-book)

Child Health and Human Development: Social, Economic and Environmental Factors
Leslie Rubin and Joav Merrick (Editors)
2013. ISBN: 978-1-62948-166-1 (Hardcover)
2013. ISBN: 978-1-62948-169-2 (e-book)

Children, Violence and Bullying: International Perspectives
Joav Merrick, Isack Kandel and Hatim A Omar (Editors)
2013. ISBN: 978-1-62948-342-9 (Hardcover)
2013. ISBN: 978-1-62948-345-0 (e-book)

Chinese Adolescent Development: Economic Disadvantages, Parents and Intrapersonal Development
Daniel TL Shek, Rachel CF Sun and Joav Merrick (Editors)
2013. ISBN: 978-1-62618-622-4 (Hardcover)
2013. ISBN: 978-1-62618-694-1 (e-book)

Chronic Disease and Disability in Childhood
Joav Merrick
2013. ISBN: 978-1-62808-865-6 (Hardcover)
2013. ISBN: 978-1-62808-868-7 (e-book)

Environmental Health Disparities in Children: Asthma, Obesity and Food
Leslie Rubin and Joav Merrick (Editors)
2013. ISBN: 978-1-62948-122-7 (Hardcover)
2013. ISBN: 978-1-62948-135-7 (e-book)

Environmental Health: Home, School and Community
Leslie Rubin and Joav Merrick (Editors)
2013. ISBN: 978-1-62948-155-5 (Hardcover)
2013. ISBN: 978-1-62948-158-6 (e-book)

Guidelines for the Healthy Integration of the Ill Child in the Educational System: Experience from Israel
Yosefa Isenberg
2013. ISBN: 978-1-62808-350-7 (Hardcover)
2013. ISBN: 978-1-62808-353-8 (e-book)

Internet Addiction: A Public Health Concern in Adolescence
Artemis Tsitsika, Mari Janikian, Donald E Greydanus, Hatim A Omar and Joav Merrick (Editors)
2013. ISBN: 978-1-62618-925-6 (Hardcover)
2013. ISBN: 978-1-62618-959-1 (e-book)

Playing with Fire: Children, Adolescents and Firesetting
Hatim A Omar, Carrie Howell Bowling and Joav Merrick (Editors)
2013. ISBN: 978-1-62948-471-6 (Softcover)
2013. ISBN: 978-1-62948-474-7 (e-book)

Promotion of Holistic Development of Young People in Hong Kong
Daniel TL Shek, Tak Yan Lee and Joav Merrick (Editors)
2013. ISBN: 978-1-62808-019-3 (Hardcover)
2013. ISBN: 978-1-62808-040-7 (e-book)

University and College Students: Health and Development Issues for the Leaders of Tomorrow
Daniel TL Shek, Rachel CF Sun and Joav Merrick (Editors)
2013. ISBN: 978-1-62618-586-9 (Hardcover)
2013. ISBN: 978-1-62618-612-5 (e-book)

Break the Cycle of Environmental Health Disparities: Maternal and Child Health Aspects
Leslie Rubin and Joav Merrick (Editors)
2013. ISBN: 978-1-62948-107-4 (Hardcover)
2013. ISBN: 978-1-62948-133-3 (e-book)

Child and Adolescent Health Yearbook 2012
Joav Merrick (Editor)
2012. ISBN: 978-1-61942-788-4 (Hardcover)
2012. ISBN: 978-1-61942-789-1 (e-book)

Child Health and Human Development Yearbook 2011
Joav Merrick (Editor)
2012. ISBN: 978-1-61942-969-7 (Hardcover)
2012. ISBN: 978-1-61942-970-3 (e-book)

Child and Adolescent Health Yearbook 2011
Joav Merrick (Editor)
2012. ISBN: 978-1-61942-782-2 (Hardcover)
2012. ISBN: 978-1-61942-783-9 (e-book)

Tropical Pediatrics: A Public Health Concern of International Proportions
Richard R Roach, Donald E Greydanus, Dilip R Patel, Douglas N Homnick and Joav Merrick (Editors)
2012. ISBN: 978-1-61942-831-7 (Hardcover)
2012. ISBN: 978-1-61942-840-9 (e-book)

Child Health and Human Development Yearbook 2012
Joav Merrick (Editor)
2012. ISBN: 978-1-61942-978-9 (Hardcover)
2012. ISBN: 978-1-61942-979-6 (e-book)

Developmental Issues in Chinese Adolescents
Daniel TL Shek, Rachel CF Sun and Joav Merrick (Editors)
2012. ISBN: 978-1-62081-262-4 (Hardcover)
2012. ISBN: 978-1-62081-270-9 (e-book)

Positive Youth Development: Theory, Research and Application
Daniel TL Shek, Rachel CF Sun and Joav Merrick (Editors)
2012. ISBN: 978-1-62081-305-8 (Hardcover)
2012. ISBN: 978-1-62081-347-8 (e-book)

Understanding Autism Spectrum Disorder: Current Research Aspects
Ditza A Zachor and Joav Merrick (Editors)
2012. ISBN: 978-1-62081-353-9 (Hardcover)
2012. ISBN: 978-1-62081-390-4 (e-book)

Positive Youth Development: A New School Curriculum to Tackle Adolescent Developmental Issues
Hing Keung Ma, Daniel TL Shek and Joav Merrick (Editors)
2012. ISBN: 978-1-62081-384-3 (Hardcover)
2012. ISBN: 978-1-62081-385-0 (e-book)

Transition from Pediatric to Adult Medical Care
David Wood, John G Reiss, Maria E Ferris, Linda R Edwards and Joav Merrick (Editors)
2012. ISBN: 978-1-62081-409-3 (Hardcover)
2012. ISBN: 978-1-62081-412-3 (e-book)

PEDIATRICS, CHILD AND ADOLESCENT HEALTH

BUILDING CHILDREN AND YOUTH FOR THE FUTURE

SOME INTERNATIONAL ASPECTS

JOAV MERRICK
ARIEL TENENBAUM
AND
HATIM A OMAR
EDITORS

nova
Medicine & Health
New York

Library of Congress Cataloging-in-Publication Data

ISBN: 978-1-53618-806-6

Published by Nova Science Publishers, Inc. † New York

CONTENTS

INTRODUCTION

In: Building Children and Youth for the Future ISBN: 978-1-53618-806-6
Editors: Joav Merrick et al.

Chapter 1

The Makor College Experience: Successes and Challenges in the First Years of a College Experience Program for Individuals with Intellectual Disability

***Stephen Glicksman*[*], PhD**
Makor Disability Services and Yeshiva University,
New York, NY, United States of America

Abstract

Recent decades have shown a tremendous increase in postsecondary education programs for college aged students with Intellectual and Developmental Disabilities. The Makor College Experience, a three year, non-degree program on the campus of a private university, is one such

[*] *Correspondence:* Adjunct Associate Professor Stephen Glicksman, PhD, Developmental Psychologist, Director of Clinical Innovation, Makor Disability Services/WLCR, 1556 38th Street, Brooklyn, 11218, New York, United States. Email: sglicksman@makords.org.

program. This chapter shares some insights that were discovered as the developers of this program attempted to overcome the challenges of including students with ID on a college campus, addressing issues such as the dialectic between being "rights-based" and "person-centered," as well as coping with the "misguided kindness" of staff and fellow students who, with the purest of intensions, tolerate inappropriate behavior of participants in the program that, in the long run, may actually hinder their growth and acceptance in the outside world.

INTRODUCTION

Recent dccades have shown a tremendous increase in postsecondary education programs for college aged students with intellectual and developmental disabilities (ID). Currently, there are close to 300 college programs for individuals with ID listed in the ThinkCollege.net database (1), in settings ranging from technical schools to large universities. Most of these programs share the samc stated purposes, and their students share the same stated goals: To provide students with ID opportunities for greater independence; to improve social skills; to develop valued social roles; and to have the normalized experience of being, "just like everyone else" (2, 3).

While being "just like everyone else" is a laudable goal, it is equally true that "everyone else" is not necessarily treated the same way across settings, nor is it true that "everyone else," even in settings aimed to promote inclusion, treat people with ID in the same way they treat their neurotypical peers. This is true in many areas, but is a particularly important variable to consider when developing programs for individuals with ID in settings where their historical exclusion is, for lack of a better term, logical. In other words, while the social and cultural experience of going to college is desired by many with ID, the exclusion of people with ID from advanced academic settings can hardly be described as "discriminatory." For that reason, inclusive postsecondary educational programs need to take into account not only the desires of the students they serve, but the realistic impact that their diagnoses may have on their social, vocational, and academic growth within the context in which the programs are being developed. The dialectic of the equally valid rights-based and person-centered approaches (5) and between equality and equity (6) should be considered when asking questions such as whether students with ID should, for example, be auditing classes with their neurotypical peers that they may be incapable of following so that they "feel like" they are in college as opposed to insisting that program participants be provided with only developmentally appropriate academic experiences in a more self-contained setting, or whether it is better to have someone with disabilities be the stereotypical water boy on the university's basketball team even if such opportunities in fact keep those with ID in the perpetual "one-down" position as opposed to supporting the individual to feel comfortable cheering the team from the stands, "just like everyone else."

With these questions in mind, we would like to share some lessons learned during the first years of a unique college experience program for individuals with ID on the campus of a private, four-year college. We begin with a brief description of the program itself, followed by a discussion of these lessons with the hope that an acknowledgment of these challenges, and how we overcame them, can serve as a model for others who hope to replicate the success of our program in their own settings.

THE MAKOR COLLEGE EXPERIENCE

Opened in the Fall of 2017, the Makor College Experience (MCE) is a three-year, non-degree, college experience program on the campus of Yeshiva University for individuals with ID. Students typically range in age from 18 to 25 years, although some students for whom this program was a "lifelong dream" began attending in their thirties. The program is a partnership between Yeshiva University and Makor Disability Services, a lifespan social services organization meeting the needs of people with intellectual and developmental disabilities since 1978. The program is technically a Day Habilitation Without Walls run by Makor Disability Services under the oversite of the New York State Office for People with Developmental Disabilities (OPWDD).

In other words, Makor Disability Services pays Yeshiva University a fee to run its program on their campus; in return, the program receives classroom and office space; access to campus resources; and the opportunity to take part and be included in campus life. The program itself mirrors a typical Yeshiva University day, which in and of itself is somewhat unique. Yeshiva University is the oldest and largest private university under Jewish auspices, and is a combination of both a modern research university and an academy of Jewish studies. The undergraduate schools of the university offer students a dual curriculum, engaging in Jewish religious studies in the morning followed by a full secular college course load in the afternoon. The MCE duplicates this model, with MCE participants engaging in self-contained classes exposing them to religious studies in the morning and secular studies in the afternoon. The afternoon classes generally focus upon life skills, liberal arts, and planning for students' futures after the program. The academic portion of the program places a heavy emphasis on vocational exploration, with Year One focusing on prevocational and job readiness skills; Year Two focusing on professionalism and off-campus career exploration outings; and Year Three focusing on concrete futures planning and resume building. Career planning is developed with the assistance of the faculty and a Vocational Coordinator based on personal interest, skills and abilities, and employment potential. A residential component to the program takes place in near-campus housing, allowing students to take full advantage of campus resources and inclusion opportunities in the evenings. MCE students are involved in student clubs; make use of the pool and gym; attend campus events; and are generally seen as fellow students by their typically developing peers. Students leave the program with a certificate of completion.

LESSONS LEARNED

Since its inception, many philosophic, educational, and legal hurdles had to be overcome, such as how to include MCE participants in student life even though they are not technically students (resolution: We have student IDs, but not student ID numbers) or how to make sure MCE participants view their own position as full-fledged members of the student community even though they are not taking classes with their college peers (resolution: Make sure MCE classes are meaningful and developmentally appropriate, and support non-academic inclusion opportunities). In overcoming these challenges, we have learned a few truths that we believe are worthwhile sharing, both for those interested in developing their own college experience programs as well as for any type of inclusive program aiming to serve people with ID in the community:

- Being real is the best way to avoid tokenism. As noted, there are currently close to 300 programs for people with specialized needs on college campuses throughout the United States (1), many in New York. Nevertheless, when representatives from OPWDD came to our program and observed our students reviewing their lessons in the student study hall; or when we pointed out a poster on the wall advertising a club that had a photo of one of our students amongst the participants; or when we pointed out how some of our third-year students are now officers student clubs; or how a college student-led initiative actually led to a change in the YU undergraduate constitution to allow our participants to vote in student elections even though, technically, they are not students; and when they saw the YU students saying, “Hi” to the Makor students by name in the hallway; the representatives commented that they had visited numerous inclusion programs on campuses, but that ours was the first that did not smack at all of “tokenism,” meaning, that the MCE students appeared to be truly included and accepted as peers. We responded that we believe that lack of tokenism is by design: We join where appropriate, and we do not where inappropriate. We do not have participants auditing college classes they cannot understand. We do not engage in activities designed to have the participants of our program “feel like” they are going to college. Rather, we designed a program that actually provides our students with a college experience, on their level, meeting their needs, as well as meeting the needs of others. We have gone so far as to call student leaders of clubs that a number of our participants were interested in joining and saying, "Be honest- how many Makor students can come to this meeting without being overwhelming to the club?" and people have been honest with us ("We can handle three- more than that would be hard"). And we, in turn, have been honest with our participants about the need to take turns or find other interests. In other words, we do our best to avoid situations where the inclusion of Makor students would most likely be viewed as a "charity," and focus on those areas in which our students are more likely to succeed as true peers. Which brings us to the second truth we have learned:

- Being real is the best way to support growth. Makor students are typically described as, "high functioning," and have had many inclusive experiences in their lives. The term "high functioning," however, is becoming somewhat controversial in some circles because it can be misleading: Makor students are "high functioning" compared to other people with ID; not, however, compared to a typical college student. The cognitive challenges of individuals described as having "mild ID" are mild compared to the rest of the population with ID; they are significantly behind the typically developing population. The social communication challenges of individuals diagnosed with Autism Spectrum Disorder are, by definition, significant, however "high functioning" a person might be viewed when compared to others with the same diagnosis. Something we realized early in our program is that the people the program was designed to serve had primarily lived inclusive lives, and, partially because of that, were used to having many of their inappropriate behaviors tolerated. They were also very used to hearing the well-intentioned but not always realistic advice that, "You can be anything you want to be." College, however, is a time to explore realistic options and to learn about one's strengths and challenges in addition to one's interests.

Because the aim of our program is to launch our graduates into meaningful, competitive jobs in the real world, we are very open, and frankly blunt, about our students' disabilities. In other words, we discovered that a primary task of our program is to help individuals develop what we refer to as an, "adaptive disability identity." It is not uncommon to hear a conversation in which a staff member tells an MCE student, "That wasn't really an appropriate way to behave," or, "That wasn't really an appropriate joke to tell," and have the student respond, "But they let me sit with them," or "But everyone laughed". The staff member will then say, "Yes, but why did they laugh? Why were they nice?" only to have the student in return smile (or not smile) and say, "Because I have Autism?" What we have learned is that almost everyone on campus will welcome our students once; but, then it is up to the students, and the staff supporting them, to have them welcomed back a second time. Part of that support is being open and honest about our students' strengths and challenges, something that we have realized many in our program have never truly experienced. That lack of experience leads, we believe, to continuing inappropriate (yet historically tolerated) behaviors, as well as unrealistic or unhealthy expectations.

One area in which this comes up frequently is employment expectations. The ultimate goal of the program is to have our students graduate with job offers, and a lot of hours are spent in the program exposing the students to different careers and work environments in an effort to expand their horizons. It is interesting to note that most students enter the program wanting to either a) do what a successful relative does, such as being a doctor or an accountant; or b) work in a school. And, in fairness, we can understand why: Because, quite often, people's dreams are limited by their experiences. In our program we often find ourselves not only trying to open the minds of our students to the wide variety of career options open to them, but equally importantly, we set up situations aimed to dissuade people from some of their current less realistic or maladaptive dreams. For example, we know that the reason many of our students want to work in school settings is because schools are an environment with which they are familiar and in which they feel safe. The reason we are not thrilled by people with ID wanting to work in school settings, however, is because we believe that in a school setting, a person with ID will always be viewed as a student and never an adult. Talking openly not just about a person's dreams and rights, but about the whole person, including his honest limitations or how he is perceived by others, and then seeing how he can expand his dreams despite those limitations and biases are what we have found helpful in leading to true growth and what has supported our students in becoming more equally welcomed, realistic, respected, and independent. Which leads to the final truth learned:

- Very well intentioned people often just don't understand. We once received a call from the head of the university's dining services, informing us that a Makor student was flirting inappropriately with staff in the dining hall. We developed a behavior plan, part of which was that the student was no longer allowed to eat in the dining hall until he showed staff that he was able to control this behavior (don't worry- there are plenty of other eateries around campus). When we informed the dining services staff of this plan, we received a response that said, "We don't mind him being here. He just requires supervision." While on its surface, this response shows a welcoming attitude on the part of the university staff, it also reflects a lack of understanding on the part of that staff to the goals of inclusion: If a person requires supervision to behave appropriately, that person is not independent. Furthermore, we believe the reason a Makor student would act in the manner this particular student did is because such behavior had been tolerated to some degree in the past due to, in this case, the person's Down syndrome. Additionally, the response of the university staff implied that this person need not be taught how to behave appropriately. Rather, he simply needed to be kept from behaving inappropriately by providing apparently lifelong supervision. So,

> while accepting his presence in the dining hall may be an example of the university staff wanting to treat this student, "just like everyone else," the fact is that "anyone else" engaging in the targeted behavior would have been banned from campus at best and arrested for sexual harassment at worst. Because of our student's Down Syndrome, in their attempt to treat our student "just like everyone else" (i.e., allowing him continued access to university facilities) the university staff were actually treating our student not only differently than everyone else in the moment, but in a manner that assumes and supports this differentiation for life (he is welcome only with supervision).

Indeed, it is not just university staff and other civilians that have difficulty with the right-based/person-centered dialectic, but even regulators and those tasked with supporting individuals with ID in the community can fall into this trap. The near-campus housing in which students of the Makor program reside is an example of this. The Makor House (as it is called) does not receive any funding from OPWDD. The reason for that is because regulations state that people with ID in new certified settings cannot reside with more than four people, as a residence with more than four individuals living communally is considered "institutional." In other words, according to current regulations, people with ID cannot live in a college dorm setting, because college dorms are institutions. This and other examples of typical college experiences not fitting into current service provision boxes is another aspect of well-intentioned people often creating barriers to actual inclusion in the name of protecting the rights of those with ID. These situations remain a paradox when developing programs that are not designed to fit neatly into current service provision paradigms.

CONCLUSION

There was a time when the greatest challenge to people with ID and the sentiments that we in the field had to fight against were those of prejudice, fear, and exclusion. Today, and definitely for the better, the sentiments we most need to fight against are misguided kindness, and inclusion as an "activity" as opposed to a reality. The challenges we have experienced in developing a college experience program for those with ID are often grounded in this idea. Nevertheless, the success of our program indicates that with forethought, honesty, and openness, these challenges can be overcome in a manner rewarding for everyone.

REFERENCES

[1] Think College. URL: https://thinkcollege.net/about/what-is-think-college.

[2] Plotner AJ, Marshall KJ. Postsecondary education programs for students with an intellectual disability: Facilitators and barriers to implementation. Intellect Dev Disabil 2015;53(1):58-69.

[3] Folk ED, Yamamoto KK, Stodden RA. Implementing inclusion and collaborative teaming in a model program of postsecondary education for young adults with intellectual disabilities. J Policy Pract Intellect Disabil 2012;9(4):257-69.

[4] Grigal M, Dwyre A, Davis H. (Transition services for students aged 18-21 with intellectual disabilities in college and community settings: Models and implications of success. Institute for Community Integration: University of Minnesota, Minneapolis, MN. NCSET Information Brief 2006;5(5).

[5] Glicksman S, Goldberg C, Hamel C, Shore R, Wein A, Wood D, et al. Rights-based and person-centered approaches to supporting people with intellectual disability: A dialectical model. Intellect Dev Disabil 2017;55(3):181-91.

[6] Piaget J. The moral judgement of the child. Harmondsworth, UK: Penguin Booksn, 1983 (First published 1932).

SECTION ONE: INTERNATIONAL ASPECTS

In: Building Children and Youth for the Future ISBN: 978-1-53618-806-6
Editors: Joav Merrick et al.

Chapter 2

A CENTURY OF MIGRATION FROM SOUTH KOREA: HISTORICAL AND DEMOGRAPHIC TRENDS

***Daniel Schwekendiek**, PhD**
Academy of East Asian Studies, Sungkyunkwan University,
Jongno-Gu, Seoul, Republic of Korea

ABSTRACT

As commonly accepted, the field of human development studies encompasses studies on both demographic wellbeing, as often indicated by mortality and morbidity, as well as on population movements, including international migration. Migration evidently falls into two categories: immigration and emigration. While immigration to South Korea is a more recent phenomenon, the nation has already experienced a century of emigration on a large scale. The purpose of this article is to provide a systematic survey on the mass "exodus" of Koreans, focusing on broad demographic trends. Methods: As North Korea and South Korea, founded in the aftermaths of World War II, are technically still at war, the two Koreas do not formally recognize each other. Thus, the

* Corresponding Author's Email: danjosch@skku.edu.

entire Korean peninsula, implying its peoples, is claimed as "property" of each respective state. A major turning point was the unexpected dissolution of the Eastern Bloc in the 1990s, enabling South Korea to add all overseas Koreans to its diaspora. Results: Official statistics put the Korean diaspora in the range of 6.6 million people in the year 2005, including 1.1 million short-term migrants. However, there was a remarkable decadal change in the number of short-term migrants from 1995 to 2005 (+295%) as a result of educational liberalization, globalization policy, and removal of emigration barriers following democratization. The remainder of this article focuses on how the "core" (long-term) Korean diasporas came into existence, arguing there were five major waves of migration. Conclusion: South Korea has emerged as one of the world's largest diaspora nations. However, permanent emigration declined by the 1990s while temporary emigration improved around that time.

INTRODUCTION

As commonly accepted, the field of human development studies encompasses studies on both demographic wellbeing, as often indicated by mortality and morbidity, as well as on population movements, including international migration (1). Migration evidently falls into two categories: immigration and emigration.

While immigration to South Korea is a more recent phenomenon, the nation has already experienced a century of emigration on a large scale. The purpose of this article is to provide a systematic survey on the mass "exodus" of Koreans, focusing on broad demographic trends.

Before addressing the state of the Korean diaspora, a discussion on diaspora-classification issues is provided through a brief historical survey.

THE STUDY

Until colonization by Japan (1910-1945), the Korean peninsula was one of the longest independent nations in the world. For instance, the preceding Goryo Dynasty (918–1392) and Joseon Dynasty (1392 to 1910) lasted for nearly a thousand years. Japan joined the Axis powers (Germany and Italy) during World War II in order to seize the opportunity to expand its territory in the Pacific. However, after two nuclear bombs were dropped on Hiroshima and Nagasaki in August 1945, the Japanese unconditionally surrendered. According to agreements reached by the Allies at diplomatic conferences held during the war, Korea was to be placed under foreign occupation. Although a four-party trusteeship (US, UK, Republic of China, and Soviet Union) was initially agreed upon by the Allies, the Korean peninsula was spontaneously split into two zones (along the 38th parallel) in the chaos of the war, with the North being occupied by the Soviets and the South by the Americans for an initial period of five years. However, due to the outbreak of the Cold War in 1947, the United Nations opted to make Korea independent earlier than planned by preparing national elections. The Soviet-backed North boycotted the elections in the South while implementing its own constitution, which led to the artificial creation of the two Koreas in 1948. Two years later, the Korean War broke out (1950-1953), ending in a stalemate that verified the previous dividing line.

It is important to note that the Korean War ended in an armistice, as no peace treaty was signed. As they are technically still at war, the two Koreas do not formally recognize each other, as shown in the constitutions of both South Korea (Article III) and North Korea (Article I). Thus, the entire Korean peninsula, implying its peoples (inside or outside of it), is claimed as "property" of each respective Korean state, and this has complicated the discussion on the diaspora immensely.

A major turning point was the thawing of the Cold War caused by the economic demise of the Soviet Union. Immediately after the political division of the Korean peninsula in 1948, the Soviet Union acknowledged the North as the legitimate and sole representative of the Korean people. However, Soviet leader and reformer Gorbachev, upon visiting South Korea in the course of the 1988 Summer Olympics hosted in Seoul, was deeply impressed by the economic success achieved by the newly industrialized South. On the other hand, South Korea pursued a policy of North-South rapprochement (*nordpolitik*) to improve its diplomatic standing and find new consumer markets. In exchange for economic support given to the Soviet Union and its satellite states, South Korea demanded its own political recognition as well as the end of subsidies to its rival in the North. The unexpected collapse of the Soviet Union and dissolution of the Eastern Bloc a few years later did not change this but even cemented the South as being recognized as the sole representative of the Korean peninsula.

The important implication of this is that South Korea has since added all overseas Koreans to its diaspora. Although North Korea does not publish any statistics on its diaspora, the South Korean government does. The data released by the South's Ministry of Ministry of Foreign Affairs and Trade suggest that the Korean diaspora more than doubled from 2.3 million in 1990 to 4.8 million in 1991 as a result of *nordpolitik* (Figure 1). In particular, addition of the large Korean diasporas in (former) communist nations such as Russia, Central Asia, and China caused this dramatic rise.

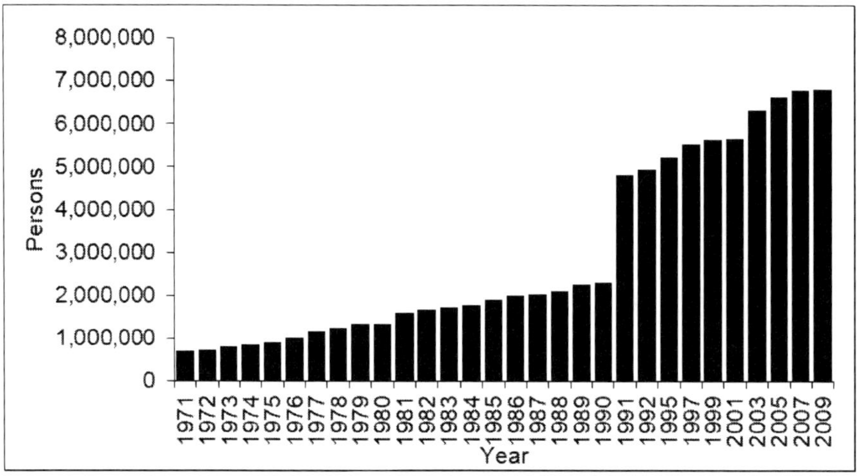

Source: Data compiled from: http://www.mofat.go.kr (accessed in 2010).

Figure 1. State of the short- and long-term Korean diaspora.

FINDINGS

Table 1 provides a survey of the state of the Korean diaspora by region. It is useful to differentiate between short-term migrants (e.g., foreign students, interns) and long-term migrants (e.g., foreign passport holders, permanent residents). Only the latter group commonly serves as an indicator of the "core" diaspora. While Figure 1 puts the Korean diaspora in the range of 6.6 million people in the year 2005, Table 1 shows that 1.1 million were short-term migrants that year. Moreover, there was a remarkable decadal change in the number of short-term migrants from 1995 to 2005 (+295%) as a result of educational liberalization, globalization policy, and removal of emigration barriers following democratization in the mid-1990s. For instance, the number of nations in which Koreans studied improved from 66 nations in 1995 to 80 nations in 2005 (2). The number of general sojourners (e.g., business visitors, working holiday visas) improved even more dramatically. Out of 1.1 million short-term migrants, about 908,000 were general (business) sojourners and 239,000 foreign students. The remainder of this article focuses on how the "core" Korean diaspora came into existence. Therefore, the focus is on long-term migrants from South Korea only (see Table 1).

Table 1. State of the long-term Korean diaspora by emigration nation, 1995-2005

Territory	Year 1995	Year 2005	Decadal change in %
China	1,926,017	2,155,664	+12
North America	1,732,273	1,823,613	+5
Japan	659,323	800,410	+21
Russian Commonwealth	459,026	523,987	+14
South America	84,963	85,515	+1
Europe	27,455	30,688	+12
Other Asia	47,775	70,293	+47
Other world	1,511	813	-46
Subtotal long-term migrants	4,938,343	5,490,983	+11
Subtotal short-term migrants	290,228	1,147,355	+295
Total	**5,228,571**	**6,638,338**	**+27**

Source: Data compiled from (3) and http://oaks.korean.net (accessed in 2010).

Similar to Japan and China, Korea was practically separated from the world through a closed-door policy in premodern times. Fishing and trade, for instance, were limited by the king to coastal waters during the Joseon period. Korea also never invaded another country over some 5,000 years of history. Lacking a global network of merchants, missionaries, and military, few Koreans made it outside of the peninsula in the past.

However, by the late nineteenth century, many farmers spontaneously traveled to Manchuria (now mostly China) and Siberia (now mostly Russia). The number of Koreans in Manchuria increased from about 8,000 people in 1860 to 200,000 in 1910, whereas the number of Koreans in Siberia improved from about 10,000 in 1882 to 45,000 in 1908 (4). On the push factor side, famine and bureaucratic corruption in the late Joseon Dynasty made many farmers seek out opportunities elsewhere since the 1860s. On the pull factor side, Manchuria and Siberia as bordering regions had lots of available fertile land. Many of these migrant farmers stayed, which partially explains the large number of Koreans in today's China and Russia (Table 1). Lacking official endorsement by any of the governments involved, this first wave of Korean emigrants can be designated as simple and spontaneous "border transgressors" (4).

The second large wave of Korean migrants was the result of Japanese colonization. Until 1905, some 7,200 Koreans were recruited to the Kingdom of Hawaii (later the United States) as sugarcane plantation farmers. However, as the Japanese seized more and more diplomatic control over the Korean peninsula even before official annexation in 1910, authorities stopped issuing passports to Koreans (5), as they could be utilized as strikebreakers against Japanese migrant workers there. This ended Korean migration to the New World, as opposed to Japanese and Chinese migration, which somehow continued through legal loopholes. More importantly, Koreans relocated in large numbers to Manchuria during colonization in order to escape Japanese authorities or to seek economic opportunities, as the Japanese seized most of the fertile plots in Korea through land reform and due to a labor shortage in the newly created Russian Maritime Province in Siberia (see below). However, after the outbreak of the second Sino-Japanese War in 1937, in which Japan invaded China, Korean migration came to a halt. Yet, from the beginning to the end of Japanese rule in Korea, the Korean diaspora in Manchuria skyrocketed from 220,000 to 1.6 million persons. More importantly, after World War II and the victory of Communism in the Chinese Civil War (1920s-1940s), Manchuria was mostly absorbed into the People's Republic of China (and the remainder into the Soviet Union). As such, Koreans could not return to North Korea, let alone to South Korea. Moreover, the Korean diaspora in China was exempted from the infamous one-child policy imposed in 1979 (though still limited to two children per family), which might in part explain its respectable growth rate (Table 1). Beyond that, Japanese colonization provided an unprecedented opportunity for Koreans to move to Japan, either as laborers or as students. After all, Japanese promoted colonial rule by emphasizing general education opportunities and civilized rule to all colonial subjects. Perhaps more importantly, Korean workers were much cheaper than local workers for Japanese employers. By 1930, as a result of the Great Depression reaching Japan, the government limited migration of Koreans, followed by an increase in Korean migration in 1939 when Japan prepared to enter World War II. Indeed, nearly 700,000 Koreans were sent to factories and mines in Japan (including Sakhalin Island, now Russia). Thus, as a result of voluntary and forced migration to Japan, the Korean diaspora in Japan improved from some 800 persons in 1910 to nearly 1.9 million persons in 1944. However, the Japanese government pressurized Koreans to leave again after World War II. Indeed, Koreans lost Japanese citizenship in 1952 (6) and a few years later also social welfare benefits, prompting many to return to South Korea, or in a some cases, to the North. It is noteworthy that although the Korean diaspora in China (at some 1.6 million) was larger than that in Japan (at some 1.9 million) at the end of World War II, the ranking positions are nowadays reversed (Table 1) for aforementioned re-migration reasons.

The third wave of Korean migration was indirectly the result of the second wave. As discussed, millions of Korean "border transgressors" arrived in Siberia and Manchuria. In the 1860s, Russia became Korea's "new neighbor" (7) by establishing the Maritime Province in the Far East, with the city of Vladivostok as the administrative center. Korean migrants living there became a part of the Russian Empire, which later became the Soviet Union. As the Korean diaspora in the Maritime Province was large in size, the Russian government always perceived it as a security threat. For instance, plans to deport Koreans to Western Siberia and Northern Russia had already been made by the beginning of the Russo-Japanese War (1904-1905) (8). Finally, Soviet leader Stalin decreed massive deportations of enemy minorities by 1937, starting with Koreans and later extending to other groups such as Germans and Turkish. Koreans were eventually deported to Russian territory in Central Asia, including today's Uzbekistan (138,000 persons), Kazakhstan (74,000 persons), and Kyrgyz Republic (3,600 persons). The large number of Koreans in the Russian Commonwealth (Table 1) is thus a combination of earlier border transgression to Siberia, migration (to Sakhalin Island and Russian parts of Manchuria) during Japanese rule, and forced deportation by Stalin in 1937.

Fourthly, Koreans were "moved by war" (9). Unlike previous migration waves taking primarily place within Asia (including Central Asia), this new wave of migrants ended up in the wealthy West. The Korean War, in which the United States entered (along with 15 other nations sending ground forces) on behalf of South Korea, resulted in a large number of civilian casualties. Some 244,000 civilians were killed, some 229,000 wounded, and some 390,000 missing, resulting in perhaps some 300,000 war widows and some 100,000 war orphans in the South (10). Korean adoptions to the United States started as a charitable mission to find new homes for countless orphans. Although Asians were generally barred from entering the United States by the Immigration Act of 1924, the Refugee Relief Act of 1953 allowed American families to adopt up to 4,000 young orphans per year until 1956 (11). After lobbying by American welfare organizations, international adoptions became enacted in United States law in 1961, thereby opening the door for mass adoptions. Following the United States, other wealthy Western nations such as Canada, France, Sweden, and Australia jumped on the bandwagon and signed international adoption agreements with South Korea. To illustrate, research suggests that two out of every three international adoptions worldwide were transacted from South Korea (12), which became the world's largest supplying nation of children in the twentieth century. In total, some 160,000 Koreans were placed for international adoption (with the vast majority arriving in the United States) by the end of the twentieth century. Note that South Korea has substantially reduced adoptions since the 1988 Olympics hosted in Seoul in order to avoid negative media coverage portraying the country as the leading "baby exporting nation". Furthermore, the War Brides Act of 1945 exempted foreign-born wives of American military personnel from the Immigration Act of 1924. Indeed, tens of thousands of American G.I.s serving in Korea during and after the war entered relationships with local women. Unlike their counterparts in West Germany or Japan (where the United States primarily set up its "empire of military bases" during the Cold War), the G.I.s stationed in South Korea were often young and unmarried. Not surprisingly, they tended to socialize with Korean women in and around camp towns. Since the beginning of the Korean War, some 100,000 Korean women have immigrated to the United States as war brides (9). Although the number of war brides is perhaps only two-thirds of that of war orphans, the former often brought their family and relatives to the United States, as a result of the Immigration and Nationality Act of 1965 which abolished the Immigration Act of 1924 discriminating against Asians. This has dramatically driven up Korean migration rates from the 1970s to 1980s. In many cases, one G.I. bride opened the door to dozens of family members, resulting in a gigantic surge of Koreans in the United States (Table 1). In addition, the new law allowed people with special skills, such as medical professionals, and those with money, such as business investors, to immigrate to the United States. Many middle class Koreans went to the United States to pursue the "American Dream" (4), especially in the 1970s and 1980s, when South Korea became more and more autocratic. As a result, Koreans became the second largest newly arriving ethnic group in the United States, following only Mexicans (13).

The fifth wave of Korean migration was caused by official contract agreements, sometimes labeled as "overseas manpower exports" (14). In fact, Korean family and business migrants of the fourth migration wave often financially supported their family back home, which might be understood as a form of labor migration. For instance, some 17% of Koreans in the United States remitted money to South Korea in 2008 (15).

However, labor migration reached a new dimension in 1962, when the new military government passed the Overseas Emigration Law (14). The law had two purposes: relieving population pressure resulting from the post-war baby boom and bringing in urgently needed foreign currency to finance the government's industrialization program. It initially targeted nations in South America such as Brazil, Argentina, Paraguay, and Bolivia through labor contract agreements. However, the program was halted in 1966 due to a lack of preparedness of the Korean settlers, even though chain migration of family members did continue. Indeed, the local governments had provided them with land to cultivate, but the majority of migrants were from urban areas in South Korea with a background in commerce and no experience in farming. In total, some 30,000 Koreans relocated to South America until 1977, explaining the relative large number of Koreans living there today (Table 1). Moreover, the government started to send contract workers to West Germany, which in turn caused the sharp rise in the number of Koreans in Europe (Table 1). As both South Korea and West Germany were nations characterized by political division (that is, one people in two countries), they engaged in mutual programs during the Cold War. In fact, West Germany was in need of workers in its post-war growth miracle years, thus opening the doors to Korean (female) nurses and (male) miners. Similar mining agreements were made with Canada and nursing agreements with Australia, although not to that extent as in the case of West Germany. In total, about 21,000 Koreans were sent to West Germany from 1962 to 1978 (4). Korean nurses alone remitted some 50 million dollars per year to South Korea (16), which represented an indispensable source of income to finance the industrialization of South Korea.

DISCUSSION

To summarize, there has been a century of mass migration from Korea. Not surprisingly, early migration was determined by geographic proximity to neighboring China, Manchuria, Russia (with many being later deported to Central Asia), and Japan. Interestingly, while mass migration of Japanese and Chinese to the New World began in the nineteenth century, few Koreans arrived in the West. However, the Korean War has "moved" many war orphans and widows to the United States. Family migration, and additionally business migration, became accelerated through a new immigration law passed in 1965. In the meantime, new forms of labor agreements with South America and especially with Germany opened the door for Koreans to enter other wealthy Western nations in the 1960s.

Interestingly, although South Korea has emerged as the world's fifth largest diaspora nation, only trailing the Chinese, Jewish, Indians, and Italians (3), emigration to major destinations such as the United States drastically declined by the 1990s. Indeed, at that time, South Korea became a fully democratized nation with an economic living standard of other industrialized nations (as evidenced by its new membership in the OECD in 1996). In the meantime, South Korea has developed itself into one of the world's fastest growing immigration countries. Alas, the latter issue is beyond the scope of the present study.

ACKNOWLEDGEMENTS

This work was supported by the Ministry of Education of the Republic of Korea and the National Research Foundation of Korea (NRF-2018S1A6A3A01023515). The authors have stated all possible conflicts of interest within this work. The authors have stated all sources of funding for this work. If this work involved human participants, informed consent was received from each individual. If this work involved human participants, it was conducted in accordance with the 1964 Declaration of Helsinki. If this work involved experiments with humans or animals, it was conducted in accordance with the related institutions' research ethics guidelines.

REFERENCES

[1] Haupt A, Kane T. Population handbook. Washington, DC: Population Reference Bureau, 1991.
[2] Weidman JC, Joh SD. Trends in the internationalization of higher education in South Korea. Int Stud Educ 2007;9:3-4.
[3] Lee K. Overseas Koreans. Seoul: Jimoondang, 2000.
[4] Kwon TH. International migration and Korean communities overseas. In: Kim DS, Kim CS, eds. The population of Korea. Daejeon: Korea National Statistical Office, 2004.
[5] Yun Y-J. Early history of Korean emigration to America (II). Korea J 1974;14:40-5.
[6] Kashiwazaki C. To be Korean without Korean nationality: Claim to Korean identity by Japanese nationality holders. In: Koh HC, Chang ET, Kim GN, King R, Ryang S, eds. Korean diaspora. New Haven, CT: Eastrock Institute, 2008.
[7] Seth M. A concise history of modern Korea: from the late nineteenth century to the present. Plymouth: Rowman Littlefield, 2010.
[8] Kim G. The deportation of 1937 as a logical continuation of Tsarist and Soviet nationality policy in the Russian Far East. In: Koh HC, Chang ET, Kim GN, King R, Ryang S, eds. Korean diaspora. New Haven, CT: Eastrock Institute, 2008.
[9] Yuh J-Y. Moved by war: migration, diaspora and the Korean War. J Asian Am Stud 2005;8:277-91.
[10] Nahm AC. Introduction to Korean history and culture. Elizabeth, NJ: Hollym, 1993.
[11] Choy CC. Institutionalizing international adoption: the historical origins of Korean adoption in the United States. In: Bergquist KJS, Vonk ME, Kim DS, Feit MD, eds. International Korean adoption: A fifty-year history of policy and practice. New York: Haworth, 2007.
[12] Huebinette T. Comforting an orphaned nation: representations of international adoption and adopted Koreans in Korean popular culture. Paju: Jimoondang, 2006.
[13] Chang ET. Korean kaleidoscope: an overview of Korean immigration to the US. In: Koh HC, Chang ET, Kim GN, King R, Ryang S, eds. Korean Diaspora. New Haven, CT: Eastrock Institute, 2008.
[14] Kim S-U. Population policies in Korea. In: Repetto R, Kwon TH, Kim SU, Kim DY, Sloboda J, Donaldson P, eds. Economic development, population policy, and demographic transition in the Republic of Korea. Cambridge, MA: Harvard University Press, 1981.
[15] Wong J, Ramakrishnan K, Lee T, Junn J. Asian American political participation: emerging constituents and their political identities. New York: Russell Sage Foundation, 2011.
[16] Schwekendiek D. Korean migration to the wealthy West. Hauppauge, NY: Nova Publishers, 2012.

In: Building Children and Youth for the Future ISBN: 978-1-53618-806-6
Editors: Joav Merrick et al.

Chapter 3

A SCOPING REVIEW OF ABUSIVE HEAD TRAUMA EPIDEMIOLOGY, LEGAL CONTROVERSIES AND PREVENTION

Debangshu Roygardner, PhD, Robert Parrish, JD, Vincent J Palusci, MD, MS and Kelli N Hughes*, JD
APSAC Center for Child Policy, Columbus,
Ohio, United States of America

ABSTRACT

Abusive head trauma (AHT) is the most common cause of morbidity and mortality due to child abuse and the most common cause of traumatic death in children less than one year old. While there has long been recognition of AHT in the medical literature, recent research has refined the scientific understanding of AHT and brought medical consensus during a concomitant increase in attention by the popular press about the legal controversies surrounding the issue. In addition, while several programs have been developed to address physical abuse or child

* *Correspondence:* Kelli N Hughes, Executive Director, APSAC Center for Child Policy, 1706 E Broad Street, Columbus, OH, 43202, United States. Email: info@centerforchildpolicy.org.

maltreatment in general, research on preventing AHT has been limited. We identified a number of empirical studies and review articles since the year 2000 and performed a scoping review to provide an overview and to synthesize the available research evidence concerning: 1) epidemiology and identification; 2) legal controversies and 3) prevention of AHT. We then suggest future directions for policy development and research in each of these areas based on the current level of scientific inquiry.

INTRODUCTION

Abusive head trauma (AHT) is the most common cause of death due to child abuse and is also the most common cause of death in children less than one year old (1). It is defined as "an injury to the skull or intracranial regions of a child under the age of five years due to blunt trauma or violent shaking" and the incidence of such may actually be an underestimation (2, 3). Indeed, some scholars indicate that the reported rates of child abuse homicide may be underreported by 50-60% (4). Survivors frequently suffer physical disabilities, neurological impairments and behavioral difficulties (5). Mortality rate estimates for AHT have been estimated at between 15%-38% and neurological morbidity for survivors is severely high (6). Often, AHT results in head trauma including intracranial hemorrhage, parenchymal injury, retinal hemorrhages and sometimes fractures of the long bones and ribs (7).

AHT includes what was described by John Caffey (1895-1978) in the 1970s as the whiplash shaken infant syndrome, later referred to simply as the shaken baby syndrome (SBS), which at that time described situations where intracranial injury was present in the absence of external signs of head trauma (8). Infants were thought to be most vulnerable to shaking given their physiology: a large head, soft neck, unmyelinated axons and a flat skull base (9). More likely than not, the perpetrator is aware that the shaking is harmful given the nature of the act (10). Other patterns of presentation include hyper-acute encephalopathy, acute encephalopathy, subdural and retinal hemorrhages, rib fracture, chronic extra-cerebral presentation and raised intra-cranial pressure (11).

Lazoritz and Bier (12) in the book "*The shaken baby syndrome: A multidisciplinary approach*" outlined its history from the earliest description until the 21st century. SBS can be traced back to 1559 with King Henri the II of France (1519-1559) who died after receiving a blow to the head during a joust. His personal physician wrote that "because of such common or shaking of the head" he died 11 days later (12). In 1946, Caffey published his landmark article "Multiple fractures in the long bones of infants suffering from chronic subdural hematoma" where he concluded that when physicians see signs of one injury (e.g., subdural hematoma) they should look for signs of another (e.g., bone fractures) which developed the concept of the medical evaluation of trauma (12). In 1968, Ayub Ommaya (1930-2008), a neurosurgeon, showed using rhesus monkeys that subdural hematoma by whiplash could be produced without impact. Caffey then built upon this assertion and the work of the British pediatric neurosurgeon Arthur Norman Guthkelch (1915-2016) to show the effects of rotational acceleration and deceleration as the etiology of subdural hematomas (12), which led to Caffey's 1972 characterization of the whiplash shaken infant syndrome.

The whiplash shaken infant syndrome became known as shaken baby syndrome. Caffey and Denver pediatrician Henry Kempe (1922-1984) also introduced the concept of the "parent-infant traumatic stress syndrome" (13, 14) which was a medical condition including non-accidental physical injury inflicted by distraught children that could include subdural hematoma and cerebral contusions. The description also included language describing the acceleration and deceleration shearing forces that produce repetitive whiplash that in turn compress the intracranial blood vessels of the brain. In 2009, the American Academy of Pediatrics recommended the use of the term "abusive head trauma" for physicians diagnosing the cause of the child's injuries, with the rationale:

> "Although shaking an infant has the potential to cause neurologic injury, blunt impact or a combination of shaking and blunt impact cause injury as well. Spinal cord injury and secondary hypoxic ischemic injury can contribute to poor outcomes of victims. The use of broad medical

> terminology that is inclusive of all mechanisms of injury, including shaking, is required." (15)

Abusive head trauma (AHT) therefore is the current nomenclature being utilized clinically and by the research field. We performed a scoping review to provide an overview of available research evidence in AHT concerning: 1) epidemiology and identification; 2) legal controversies; and 3) prevention. We searched PubMed, Google Scholar, and PsychINFO for articles and other materials related to these topics published since the year 2000 and synthesized the research to suggest future directions for research and policy development in each of these areas based on the current level of scientific inquiry.

EPIDEMIOLOGY AND IDENTIFICATION

Differentiating between AHT and non-abusive head trauma can be difficult despite some clear differences in patient presentation and case history (16). A large proportion of AHT patients may be initially misdiagnosed, underdiagnosed or diagnosed too late to prevent injury (5). 31.2% of AHT cases were found by Jenny et al. (16) to be missed at initial presentation, and 28% of children were later re-injured, indicating a clear need for improved recognition of signs for AHT. Niederkrotenthaler, Xu, Parks and Sugerman (5) conducted a descriptive study on the socio-demographic data of children who had been diagnosed with AHT. In this four-year study, rates of AHT per 100,000 were higher in children under one year old, males and Blacks; more of the AHT cases were fatal (6.7%) as opposed to fatal cases in the nonabusive head trauma group (1.8%). Cases that were covered by public insurance or were uninsured had increased odds of being diagnosed with AHT. Given that insurance status is a good predictor of socio-economic status, the risk of AHT was associated with socio-economic disadvantage, making them more at risk (5). Similarly, AHT and its relationship to economic hardship was explored by Wood et al. (17) in an investigation of the link between the economic recession and AHT. The authors found that the rate of AHT increased during the recession, providing further evidence for the relationship between parental stress and violence. The lifetime cost of AHT based on one single year (2010) was $13.5 billion with an estimated breakdown of $257 million for medical care, $552 million for special education, and $322 million for child protective services and criminal justice costs. (18). Peterson, Xu, Florence and Parks (19) estimated the medical costs of AHT among patients 0-4 years over a 5-year period to be $69.6 million nationwide for hospital visits alone.

Scribano, Makoroff, Feldman and Berger (20) studied the characteristics of perpetrators of AHT over a five-year period. Alleged perpetrators were more likely to be fathers (53%), followed by parent partner (22%), mother (8%), babysitter (8%) and other adult caregiver (5%). Non-parental perpetrators were more likely to cause head injury to a child over the age of 1y, suggesting that some interventions need to focus as well on the post infancy age. Gender differences between male and female perpetrators have also been explored (21) and have shown significant perpetrator differences. The median age for female perpetrators (34y) was higher than for males (27y) and male perpetrator gender was associated with worse clinical outcomes, surgical intervention, perpetrator confession, and criminal conviction. Children with a male perpetrator were much more likely to suffer worse outcomes, even death. Parental risk factors for abuse include substance abuse, domestic violence, criminal history, unrealistic expectations and attachment problems (22).

Perpetrator confessions have also been examined to see if they correlate with mechanisms of injury (23). Shaking was described as extremely violent in 100% of the cases and was repeated in 55% of the cases, with the mean number of times shaken being 10. The majority of confessions indicated that shaking was done to stop infant crying (62.5%), and impact was not used. Another study of perpetrator confessions by Biron and Shelton (24) indicates that perpetrator accounts described an immediate neurological response from the victim, suggesting that the symptoms of head injury were immediately notable.

Key elements in the identification of AHT

AHT is a difficult area to study and presents several methodological concerns. The scholars and scientists in the extant literature tended to follow two general methods (25). Outcomes may be analyzed through observation of incidents of AHT with comparison to known accidental injuries, and researchers can extrapolate to identify patterns. Otherwise, researchers can develop experimental animal or biomechanical models of different types of traumas and then scale these to AHT with regard to infants (25). Another method is to use meta-analysis of the extant literature of one or the other category just highlighted.

The first breakthrough in the biomechanics of head trauma came from Athelstan Hylas Stoughton Holbourn (1907-1962) (26), a British physiologist who began to identify and analyze the forces required for cerebral injury. He made five assumptions about the brain: that it had uniform density, that it was about as incompressible as water, that it could change shape easily in response to an applied force, that the skull was more rigid than the brain, and that the shape of the brain and the size of the head mattered when it came to cerebral injury. Holbourn (26) noted that rotational shearing forces were critical in producing concussive symptoms and significant brain injury.

Caffey (8) found that subdural hematoma and cortical injury found in infants were similar to the shear strain hypothesis identified by Holbourn (26) and that it also represented what looked to be a whiplash phenomenon. During this period, scholars postulated that rotational acceleration was critical in the pathogenesis of brain injury in abused infants in comparison to those seen in short falls (25). Ommaya, Faas and Yarnell (27) added to this body of literature in an experimental study examining adult monkeys and chimpanzees. Ommaya and colleagues proposed critical tolerances based on shearing forces for concussion, subdural hematoma and diffuse axonal injury in humans. Work by Gennarelli et al. (28) found that the development of diffuse axonal injury was due to the duration of trauma in addition to the axis of rotation, with more prolonged and coronal rotation likely to lead to subdural hematomas.

He and his colleagues identified the metabolic changes in axonal membranes and micro-glia after rotational trauma.

Several other descriptive factors have been found in infants with AHT. Moving to a design with controls, Imagawa et al. (29) compared 17 infants with a diagnosis of AHT with a control sample. Results indicated that reduced axonal diffusivity was shown in widespread white matter regions in the AHT infants and that these findings related to a worse prognosis and clinical outcomes. Work by Narang and Clarke (30) identified subdural and retinal hemorrhages as most common findings in AHT. The authors defined subdural hemorrhage as a traumatic hemorrhage developed from torn veins between the brain and the dural sinus as opposed to other theories, which historically proposed they emerged from illnesses. Narang and Clarke (30) further posit that infants with AHT suffer from an array of symptoms that can range from non-specific (i.e., irritability, poor feeding and vomit) to delayed development to life-threatening conditions such as respiratory compromise and seizures.

Cervical spine injury may also be an underreported aspect of AHT; initial studies indicated a low detection rate in children with confirmed inflicted trauma (35%) however more recent studies have shown the rate to be as high as 44% (30). Some other manifestations include spinal cord injury with ligament injury, fractures, or spinal cord injury without radiologic abnormality. In the cases where an infant survived AHT, they often developed epilepsy, severe neurological impairment, motor and visual deficits, sleep disorders, language abnormalities and attention and behavioral disorders (31).

Piteau, Ward, Barrowman and Plint (32) conducted a meta-analysis of 24 studies from 2000-2009 to determine the differences between clinical and radiological variables of AHT as opposed to non-abusive head trauma. Their results indicated that "subdural hemorrhages, cerebral ischemia, retinal hemorrhages, skull fractures, metaphyseal fracture(s), long bone fracture(s), rib fracture(s), seizure(s), apnea, and no adequate history given" were significantly associated with AHT (32). In comparison, epidural hemorrhage, scalp swelling, and isolated skull fracture were significantly associated with non-AHT. Subdural hemorrhages (SDH) have been reported in 77%-90% of AHT patients, and retinal hemorrhages have been reported in 74%-82% (30). Multiple subdural hemorrhages and those within the interhemispheric fissure and over the convexities were related to AHT in a statistically significant way. Shein et al. (33) conducted a quasi-experimental study on risk factors that then predicted mortality in infants with AHT. Their analysis included 386 children with AHT, and their findings indicated that a low score on the Glasgow Coma Scale, retinal hemorrhage, intraparenchymal hemorrhage and cerebral edema were independently associated with mortality.

Intracranial injuries, rib fractures, and retinal hemorrhages (RH) are the most common physical findings predictive of AHT (34-37). Much of this literature also borrows from experimental methods used with piglets that were shown to have ocular hemorrhage in 73%, including in the anterior chamber, vitreous and optic nerve (35). Retinal hemorrhages are the most common ophthalmological finding in AHT and are estimated at 85% prevalence (36). RH tend to occur more frequently in children who die than those who survive and have a low incidence in child abuse by blunt trauma only or short falls. In cases of severe accidental head trauma, the incidence is usually between 0-3%. Maguire et al. (37) found that RH were found in 78% of AHT versus 5% of non-AHT, and that, in a child with head trauma and RH, the probability for abuse is 91%. Highly numerous and multi-layered RH are highly specific for AHT (36). They are not likely to be explained by a differential diagnosis of hypoxia alone since they do not occur in other disorders with cerebral hypoxia. Retinal folds and traumatic retinoschisis are also highly specific for AHT; indeed, in one meta-analysis, no studies documented retinal folds or retinoschisis in conditions other than AHT (36, 38). Other studies have shown that RH were bilateral in 83% of AHT cases in comparison to 8.3% in non-AHT, with a few RH located in the posterior pole and only 10% extending to the periphery in non-AHT (37). A different study found that severe, multi-layered RH were only seen in 3.7% of patients without AHT (e.g., leukemia and sepsis, illness during birth) (34).

Scientists in varied fields, medical practitioners and researchers over the past sixty years have contributed to the knowledge base for the identification of AHT. The science has moved forward to better understand the symptoms and radiologic factors associated with AHT and to more correctly and effectively identify the diagnosis. As with all medical diagnoses, the collective experience of those who regularly diagnose the cause, timing and mechanism of childhood head injuries is enhanced by research findings and has resulted in significant clinical advancements (39). In a synthesis of the science to date, four recommendations emerge with the potential to influence policy at the intersection of practice and research: (1) practitioners should utilize a multi-disciplinary team to focus on symptoms with high specificity and predictive validity as determined by the literature in order to make diagnoses with confidence; (2) practitioners should seek immediate ophthalmological consultation if a child is being assessed for head trauma; (3) the field needs to develop more prospective, controlled studies using commonly accepted definitions for terms; and (4) the field needs to enhance bio-mechanical models to most appropriately reflect the anatomy and physiology of the human infant.

LEGAL DISAGREEMENTS AND CONTROVERSIES

Overall, approximately 1,500 people are involved in the legal system annually regarding some form of AHT or SBS in the US, and approximately 200 people per year are prosecuted and convicted (40). In the criminal court system, about 40% of AHT cases result in prosecution with a conviction rate of 88%, although AHT and SBS per se are not listed specifically in the definitions of crimes (4). There are legal disagreements in the literature regarding the diagnosis of AHT. Legal defenders often believe that many individuals charged and convicted of AHT are actually innocent, while prosecutors often believe that many guilty perpetrators go free, thus "compromising society's responsibility to protect infants from abuse" (4).

Overall, ethical citizens on either the prosecution or defense side of the legal debate would not want to see an innocent person go to jail nor would they want to see a guilty person go free. All want children protected and parents' rights appropriately preserved. But it appears that, despite the 40 years of evidence in the field and the more than 1,000 peer-reviewed articles supporting the AHT diagnosis, there continues to be inconsistencies within the judicial system regarding the use of the diagnosis. What is of considerable concern is that different AHT cases with similar findings have led to disparate court verdicts, often with inconsistent sentencing, ranging from going free, to probation, to life in prison. Much of what drives these differences may be due to expert witnesses, some of whom have "variable credentials" and may use unique interpretations of medical evidence to make the jury feel that there is enough confusion to create "reasonable doubt" (4).

Some legal scholars argue that AHT or the shaken baby syndrome diagnosis are unproven hypotheses which do not meet admissibility frameworks in national and international courts (40-43). Slovis, Strouse, Coley and Rigsby (44) recognized that some child abuse "denialists" have even falsely claimed that the diagnosis of AHT or child abuse is "the creation of a non-disease." Defense-biased law professors and law students have published legal articles claiming that the issue of AHT is the "next innocence project" (41). Others have argued simply that there is scant "evidence-based medical or empirical evidence on that issue (42, 43). These legal arguments have been refuted (44-48).

According to Gabaeff (49), there is a medical controversy in child abuse pediatrics between "an established corps of child abuse pediatricians aligned with hospital colleagues and law enforcement, and a multi-specialty challenger group of doctors and other medical professionals working with public interest lawyers." He goes on to state that "as the ability to convict based on this unproven prime hypothesis, that subdural hemorrhage plus retinal hemorrhage equals abuse, some defense attorneys were professionally compelled … to seek second opinions" (49). Gabaeff appears to be one of a small group of physicians who deny the existence or prevalence of child abuse, testify in courtrooms as to unproven alternative explanations for inflicted childhood head injuries, and regularly try to confuse the triers of fact in child abuse litigation. Some claimed controversies in the area focus on issues related to lucid intervals, rebleeding of chronic subdural hematomas, alternate theories of explanation including hypoxia and short falls causing death, and a claim that the shaken baby syndrome has been abandoned by mainstream medical diagnosticians. Unfortunately, there are "unethical and unqualified" physicians whose testimony may be described as irresponsible according to legal and medical rules of ethics who nevertheless continue to propagate unfounded and scientifically unproven claims which represent unusual interpretations of medical findings, but which have led to hung juries and acquittals and even appellate court reversals of prior convictions or granting of new trials based on the claim of "new science" not available at the time of trials (50).

Those who believe that AHT is "unproven" state that the scientific proof boils down to three essential features known as "the triad" which include subdural hematoma, retinal hemorrhages, and acute encephalopathy (40). Tuerkheimer (41) also discusses "the triad" as now being undermined by current research, and that the triad can no longer be seen as "pathognomonic of AHT." This claim that a triad of findings automatically results in a diagnosis of abusive head trauma has never been accurate, yet it is accepted uncritically by those who desire to deny the existence of child abuse. It was originally coined by child abuse denialists as a "straw man" foil for their arguments but is akin to the specious claim of legal writers that a diagnosis of AHT is a legal "diagnosis of murder." Henneberg (43) indicates that the "triad … is not reliable" and that courts ought to pay more attention to the advances in scientific thinking. Few articles include the term "triad" in their description of AHT, yet the concept continues to be a popular term in the popular press (51) and legal journals such as the Oklahoma City University of Law Review (40) and the Washington University Law Review (42).

It is beyond the capacity of this scoping review to outline every single alleged controversy present in the field of AHT. However, three themes emerge: 1) whether studies are scientifically rigorous, generally accepted, and meet the criteria for admissibility in U.S. courts (52); 2) alternate theories that better explain the injuries a child suffered which range from paroxysmal coughing, vomiting, to the "unified hypothesis" of hypoxia and raised venous pressure and other conditions which potentially “mimic” the symptoms seen in AHT (52-54); and, 3) the argument that AHT is essentially “medical diagnosis of murder” in that all three components of who, when, and intent are answered through one diagnosis and one expert witness, allegedly circumventing the legal process (40, 42). These assertions have received substantial medical and legal responses (55, 56).

Are these studies scientific enough?

Ultimately, it is unethical to randomly sort infants into abuse and non-abuse groups in order to conduct randomized, prospective controlled experiments to determine causation of childhood head injuries. Therefore the closest proxies (whether they be bio-mechanical models or scaling of animals such as pigs or woodpeckers) are sometimes inappropriately claimed to be biofidelic indicators of the thresholds for human child head injury. Thus, Geddes and Whitwell (53) indicate that in their study of the literature “there have been no systematic formal neuropathological studies of infant head injury” and that the “evidence base for diffuse axonal injury being a common finding in infant head injury is poor.” Gabaeff (49) indicates that the theory on AHT essentially follows the same pattern of thought – that “a caregiver snapped under stress,” they then shook a child in an abusive manner, and was then assumed to be guilty. Gabaeff goes on to indicate that studies indicate the improbability of the “snapping” hypothesis and the probability of a previously caring caregiver “snapping” is less than 1/10,000. Gabaeff continues to make other arguments critical of the “shaking hypothesis” including that current biomechanical testing indicates that humans could not produce shearing forces strong enough to cause brain damage (without also causing neck injury), that observational methods have been used in most studies (which is not an evidence based methodology), that researchers use a circular logic in these observational studies, and that multi-disciplinary teams in hospitals are prone to “group-think” that thereby derides their ability to operate as objective scientists.

Findley et al. (40) also claim that when doctors began applying "evidence-based medicine" standards that required "biostatistical significance" and the scientific method, most of the research on AHT did not meet the "quality under evidence based medicine standards." Furthermore, they allege that the majority of the AHT cases fall to the bias of the "prosecutors fallacy," the notion that the researchers "ignored the base rate," that is to say that the researchers did not look at the rate at which abuse is present compared to all of the cases of infant death. Finally, they posit that research for AHT suffer from selection bias, observer bias or both in that the validity of the research depends on whether researchers are accurately identifying which cases reflect abuse and which do not, since often "the very diagnostic signs that are used to sort the cases into these two categories are the same signs that the studies are purporting to measure."

Researchers who support the generally accepted diagnosis of AHT assert on the contrary that much of the alternate research is based on case reports and circular logic; some even go as far as to say that omissions and misrepresentations are made (57). Indeed, sometimes case reports are made by authors involved in defense litigation who have never treated the child, and which often diverge with sworn testimonies. Jenny (58) indicates that "the evidence base supporting many of the explanations offered to disprove abusive head trauma is often quite weak" and that in the case of suspected accidental trauma, a thorough workup is required to improve accurate diagnosis. Hymel et al. (59) outlined a 10-step process in ruling out differential diagnoses in order to make the appropriate diagnosis of AHT; some of these steps include paying close attention to the clinical presentation of the child in addition to consultation with radiologists and appropriate radiological exams.

Alternate theories and their shortcomings

In Geddes et al. (60), 53 cases of non-accidental head injury were subjected to detailed neuro-pathological study. Results indicated that the most usual cause of death was raised intracranial pressure secondary to brain swelling in 82% of the cases and that hypoxic brain damage was present in 77% of the cases. Furthermore, diffuse axonal injury was present in only 3/53 cases. Geddes and Whitwell (54) provide a separate hypothesis than what they deem the "traditional explanation" which includes injury to the child yielding bruising and skull fracture, in addition to brain swelling, subdural and retinal hemorrhage. They indicate that their hypothesis does not necessarily emanate from injury, it could also be due to genetic susceptibility, which could lead to apnea, severe hypoxia, brain swelling and then subdural and retinal bleeding. Geddes and Whitwell (54) indicate that intracranial bleeding may be "a phenomena resulting from deranged infant physiology rather than a direct result of trauma" and that "such a possibility highlights the difficulty of being certain that abuse has occurred in cases where there is no objective evidence of trauma or violence."

Other alternate theories not discussed before include: that normal, healthy infants suddenly die after birth because a birth related hematoma spontaneously rebleeds, that subdural hemorrhages in infants are caused by immunizations, and that short falls can cause the same signs and symptoms of abusive head trauma (58). Despite these alternate theories, Albert et al. (4) indicate that most physicians treating AHT agree that these cases can be diagnosed or "ruled out" on the basis of routine diagnostic or follow up studies. According to Albert et al. (4), the issue arises when some defense lawyers choose to present an isolated portion of medical findings rather than the totality of all medical findings in order to "confuse the jury." Furthermore, the presentation of such complex medical information itself presents a problem in that expert witnesses have to explain the material in a clear and understandable way to the judge and jury (4). Although the list of alleged alternative explanations offered in the courtroom is long, none of them have been proven through valid empirical research to explain the collection of head, eye and other injuries which are part of the diagnosis of AHT.

Given this backdrop, several authors who actually are experts in the field of child maltreatment have accurately characterized the "debate" over the shaken baby syndrome or abusive head trauma as a "legal" debate, not a serious scientific debate. Within the relevant scientific fields of those who regularly diagnose the cause of infant and toddler injuries, almost all accept AHT and SBS as valid diagnoses and reject the alternative theories offered by the child abuse "denialists" (61). In his article "Child abuse: We have problems," Dr Peter Strouse (62) makes a persuasive case that child abuse denialism "has at its base a very small number of physicians who perpetuate false science while ignoring the bulk of the scientific literature and the experience of the overwhelming majority… The names are familiar, they reference one another in the literature and they show up in court, often together and all too frequently… The denialists create the appearance of scientific and medical controversy when, in almost all cases, there is none. Rather than providing clarification, the denialists' tactics are to confuse judges and jurors, to bias the news media and to mislead the public." In "*Understanding abusive head trauma in infants and children: Answers from America's pediatricians,*" child abuse pediatrician Dr Cindy Christian (63) clarifies the position of the American Academy of Pediatrics that both shaken baby syndrome and abusive head trauma are well-accepted legitimate diagnoses, stating: "There is no legitimate medical debate amount the majority of practicing physicians as to the existence or validity of AHT/SBS. The only real debate and controversy appear to be in the legal system and the media." While some have offered alternative hypotheses in the courtroom, "the evidence for these hypotheses is lacking." Dr Christian concluded by refuting the validity of many of the courtroom claims of the child abuse denialists and pointing out there are well over 1000 articles in the peer-reviewed clinical literature supporting the diagnoses of SBS/AHT (63).

A recent consensus statement on abusive head trauma in infants and young children, endorsed by the American Academy of Pediatrics, American Professional Society on the Abuse of Children, the Society for Pediatric Radiology and other international societies summarized the various unsubstantiated theories which are used to explain pediatric SDH or AHT (55, 64). They noted that: 1) cerebral sino-venous thrombosis (CSVT) represents a serious disorder with high rates of morbidity and mortality; however, reviews of large pediatric studies of CSVT have failed to show the connection between CSVT and SDH; 2) hypoxic ischemic injury theory (HII) proposed by Geddes et al. (55) was tested by comparing HII alone with HII along with AHT, and no SDH was identified in the non-traumatic HII cohort (65); 3) there is currently no body of medical evidence to support the hypothesis that SDH following lumbar puncture causes all the findings of AHT; 4) although one case study has shown dysphagic choking as a hypothesis (66), recent studies do not support this assertion (67); and 5) benign enlargement of the subarachnoid space (BESS) causes few SDH without trauma since, out of 712 reported cases of BESS, only 1.7% represented subdural collections that were hemorrhagic in nature, and many (41.7%) were hemorrhagic due to accidental trauma or abuse (68).

The fallacy of the 'diagnosis of murder'

Some have made legal arguments that the diagnosis of AHT is equivalent to the "medical diagnosis of murder" that circumvents the traditional legal processes in determining levels of intent (41). However, it has been pointed out that medical practitioners do not diagnose "murder." While forensic pathologists and coroners may list *homicide* as a manner of death on death certificates, the Consensus Statement (55) concluded that the diagnosis of AHT is a medical diagnosis made by a multidisciplinary team of pediatricians and pediatric subspecialty physicians, social workers and other professionals based on consideration of all the facts and findings, and that AHT is a scientifically non-controversial medical diagnosis broadly recognized and managed throughout the world. Furthermore, it states that: "Given that medical findings do not identify the perpetrator or intent required for *murder*, a diagnosis of AHT is a medical conclusion, not a legal determination of the intent of the perpetrator or, in the false hyperbole of the courtroom and sensationalistic media, not a diagnosis of murder."

PREVENTION

While the research included in our review reflects a small but relatively strong collection of studies about programs specifically designed to prevent AHT, well-designed outcome evaluations are sparse but increasing. Lopes and Williams (69) found a total of 1,215 articles over 10 years addressing AHT prevention, but only 34 were deemed eligible for study since the remainder were duplicative, non-empirical, pre-2005, unavailable or did not address prevention. Moreover, most studies are of AHT prevention are observational, and, even when randomized controlled trials have been used in the field of child abuse in general, there are often too many methodological limitations to draw reliable conclusions as to their effectiveness in AHT prevention (70). Despite this, there have been several attempts that focus on screening, professional education, parental education within the context of medical settings, and prevention programs which focus on infant crying as a trigger.

Screening tools for AHT

Letson et al. (71) examined the number of opportunities that medical or child protective staff had for identifying and referring a child with symptoms consistent with abuse. Authors found that 31% of their patients surveyed had a prior opportunity of having their abuse identified, and 25% had one prior opportunity in a medical setting. They found no differences in age, gender, race or insurance status. The most common prior opportunities within the medical setting included chronic subdural hemorrhage and healing fractures in addition to vomiting, prior CPS contact and bruising (71). Other concerns for missed AHT include "sentinel injuries" defined as certain previous injuries in the medical history that were suspicious. Sheets et al. (72) found that in a sample of 200 abused infants, 27.5% had previously had a sentinel injury as opposed to none of the 101 non-abused infants. The most common form of sentinel injury in the abused cohort was bruising (80%); sentinel injuries tended to occur early in infancy with 95% occurring before the age of 7 months (72).

One concern with prevention programming is the potential impact of screening on the reduction of AHT. Bailhache, Bénard and Salmi (73) studied the impact of screening tools, with the potential side effects being that parents could be wrongfully accused of being an abuser. Their research indicated that after a two-year period, the median number of deaths avoided ranged from 6 to 28 per 100,000 newborns (73). The overall impact of the screening process was determined to be uncertain. Hymel, Herman, Narang, et al. (74) developed a validated clinical screening tool for the identification of AHT. Their results suggest that their AHT screening tool could increase AHT detection in the pediatric intensive care unit setting from 87% to 96% and increase the overall diagnostic yield of completed evaluations from 49%-56% while targeting less children for evaluation. Another screening tool developed by Cowley, Morris, Maguire et al. (75), known as the PredAHT (Predict AHT), also showed promise, with a sensitivity of 72.3% and a specificity of 85.7% and an AHT estimation probability of 81.5%. Six features were recorded in the screen scale, including retinal hemorrhage, rib and long bone fractures, apnea, seizures, and head and neck bruising.

Evidenced informed and evidence based education programs

Education programs have shown varying levels of empirical evidence for their effectiveness. Some parents are not aware of AHT or the dangers associated with it (76), leading to evaluation of parent education strategies. One study (76) found that 27% of mothers and 36% of fathers had never heard of AHT, and a brief talk by medical staff was useful in increasing their knowledge. Going one step further, Altman et al. (77) evaluated the effectiveness of a leaflet and 8-minute video explaining AHT. Pre-post analysis indicated that there was a 75% reduction in injuries in the year after the training program was introduced. Some of these programs have been evaluated in an international context, and programs that were developed in the United States have used international replication studies for empirical cross-cultural validation. For example, in Turkey, an educational film was utilized as a prevention program and outcomes suggested that the average levels of knowledge increased over time with the most effective learning time occurring prior to birth and three to seven days after birth (78).

Infant crying has been widely regarded as one trigger for abuse. Perpetrators may lack sufficient knowledge, relationship skills and/or impulse control to manage infant behaviors. Prolonged, unsoothable crying in early months has been interpreted in various ways including pathology with the infant, pathology with the caregiver or a pathological interaction between the two. Barr (79) interpreted the increase in the proclivity for violence during infant crying as a breakdown in the normative dynamics of the infant-caregiver relationship, and he recommends strategies aimed at educating adults regarding the normative development curves of infants and how to respond appropriately. The *"Period of Purple Crying"* is considered an evidence based model that has been subject to a randomized control trial in addition to independent replication (80, 81). [The letter PURPLE each stand for a property of the types of crying that frustrates caregivers: P for peak, U for unexpected, R for resistance, P for pain-like look, L for long bouts, and E for evening (80)]. Another study showed that new mothers found the program useful in teaching them about normal infant crying and soothing and coping strategies (82).A randomized, controlled trial with 1279 mothers showed statistically significant improvements in knowledge and self-reports of walking away when the child is inconsolable. A cross-cultural replication study in Japan showed knowledge scores and self-reported walking away behavior that were significantly higher in the intervention group (81). Another study reported that such an evidence-based education program may be successful in reducing the incidence of AHT during an economic recession (83).

Dias et al. (84) used a hospital-based prevention program where nursing and medical staff were asked to provide mothers and fathers information describing the dangers of infant shaking, including providing alternative parenting strategies. Both parents were asked to sign a voluntary 'commitment statement' to never shake their child and to inform any others caring for their child about the dangers and to get a commitment from them. The methods included a quasi-experimental, retrospective longitudinal design which showed that incidences of child maltreatment after the introduction of the prevention program decreased 47%. Limitations of the study include that it was not a randomized control trial and that the results did not follow a dose response pattern. Kelly et al. (85) did an independent cross-cultural replication also using a quasi-experimental design in New Zealand on a sample of 2,592 caregivers. Results indicated that 85% of respondents remembered one key message from the intervention and that 92% made a plan of what to do when frustrated. Interestingly, the results were statistically significant despite the lack of commitment statements that were hypothesized to be a key determinant of success in the original study (84).

Morrill et al. (86) implemented and evaluated a media-based program called *"All Babies Cry"* that focused on reducing parental stress and soothing infants. Results indicated that, after 17 weeks, the intervention group of used a wider variety of skills than did the control group and reported using stress reduction strategies depicted in the program.

Others have focused on the education of primary healthcare providers. One such model is the SEEK program which also meets the criteria for evidenced-based. The SEEK model includes the training of child health care primary care professionals, a parent questionnaire which screens for potential problems, and a "reflect-empathize-assess-plan" approach to address the problems identified in the screening (87). Two large randomized control trials were conducted – one in a resident training clinic serving low income, African American families, and the other in 18 suburban pediatric private practices serving middle income, mostly White families (87, 88). In the first study, SEEK children were significantly less likely to be maltreated, including fewer CPS reports, fewer documented incidences of medical neglect, and fewer instances of severe physical assault reported by parents. In the second, SEEK mothers reported fewer minor physical assaults than controls at 6 months and 12 months follow up.

Other programs have utilized partnerships between healthcare providers and services in the home setting. Donelan-McCall, Eckenrode and Olds (89) assert that over the past twenty years, one of the most effective means of preventing child maltreatment has come from health services and parenting education within the home since several of these programs have shown empirical promise. The Nurse Family Partnership Program (NFP) pioneered by David Olds and begun in Elmira, NY using nurse home-visitors, was tested in a randomized, control trial and showed 80% fewer cases of abuse in the intervention group. NFP was also replicated in Memphis, TN in a trial which showed that children in the control group were 4.5 times more likely to have died from child maltreatment than were their counterparts in the intervention group. Another program using non-nurse home visitors, *Hawaii Healthy Start*, was evaluated, and no effect was found on child abuse and neglect (90). A key element determining effectiveness has been postulated to be the professional status and experience of the home visitors.

One particularly promising form of prevention is the community based *Strong Communities for Children* (SCC) program (91, 92). SCC is a comprehensive community-wide initiative that promotes a narrative change in the perceptions, beliefs and behavior of community members (92). Implementation includes the phases of "spreading the word," "mobilizing the community," "increasing resources for families" and "institutionalizing resources." Three related studies using random sampling were compared to a comparison sample, and results indicate moderate effect sizes for both coded child injuries and founded cases of abuse and neglect. These studies are promising on two fronts: 1) the measure the actual outcome of child abuse itself rather than scaling from self-reports or intentions for harm, and 2) effect sizes which are in the moderate range.

Other strategies to measure effective implementation are in the literature. One is the *RE-AIM* ("reach, adoption, implementation and maintenance") framework, which has been used to evaluate statewide implementation of AHT prevention programs (93). Using it, 86 state hospitals were able to implement the program with high fidelity, and the majority were able to incorporate the program into unit procedures and employee training, with a majority of hospitals indicating their desire to continue the program into the future.

NEXT STEPS

There are several questions that need to be answered through further research to inform our prevention strategies and influence policy and practice. Even though science has developed considerably over the past 20 years, there is still far to go if we are to achieve effective AHT identification and prevention (94). It is also unclear whether general community monetary supports will affect risk for child maltreatment, or whether child maltreatment prevention programs in general will address AHT specifically. For example, should certain conditions immediately be followed by protocols in hospitals? (e.g., children found with sentinel wounds immediately have caregiver referred to AHT prevention). Given that the science behind screening tools is strong, medical and para-medical professionals should be trained on these and the results measured.

Legal controversies will prompt a different response. A recent review concluded that, with a commitment of practitioners to apply the best medical science and of lawyers to become more knowledgeable and to articulately educate judges and jurors, we can expose the inaccurate testimony of irresponsible medical witnesses and mitigate the effects of legal misunderstandings and subterfuge (56). Thus more research will be needed to assess whether courts, lawyers and jurors can be affected by policy or practice with a collective multi-disciplinary focus that addresses not only the need for better AHT identification among the general public, but also exposing flawed media coverage of the topic. Given that one-sided media coverage may focus on flawed claims that the shaken baby syndrome is no longer accepted by mainstream diagnosticians, it is not dangerous to shake infants and toddlers, or that caretakers have been falsely accused of abusing their children, successful prevention efforts may need to evaluate public media and strategies that begin by neutralizing public misperceptions.

While prevention science is most mature in the areas of parent education and home visiting, there is wide variability in efficacy. Non-significant findings noted in many studies of prevention strategies indicate the need to better identify the groups for whom such strategies can be effective as well as better means to reach high risk families contributing to AHT rates. Additional research will need more sophisticated methods and randomized controlled trials, but there are ethical concerns regarding randomization. For home visiting, questions remain regarding who best provides the service, which populations are better served, and whether it effects AHT or child maltreatment in general. We have suggested that many or all of these strategies can be combined in community-based *prevention zones* that are directed at decreasing all forms of child maltreatment, including AHT (95). While more research is also needed to understand parent behavior, professional practice, and social and community factors, a more broad and universal approach in all of these areas of focus needs to be comprehensive, accepted, and available for everyone at the community level.

REFERENCES

[1] Bechtel K, Stoessel K, Leventhal JM, Ogle E, Teague B, Lavietes S, Duncan C. Characteristics that distinguish accidental from abusive injury in hospitalized young children with head trauma. Pediatrics 2004;114(1):165-8.

[2] Parks SE, Annest JL, Hill HA, Karch DL, eds. Pediatric abusive head trauma: Recommended definitions for public health surveillance and research. Atlanta, GA: Centers for Disease Control and Prevention, 2012.

[3] Kelly P, Thompson JM, Koh J, Ameratunga S, Jelleyman T, Percival TM, Mitchell EA. Perinatal risk and protective factors for pediatric abusive head trauma: A multicenter case-control study. J Pediatr 2017;187:240-6.

[4] Albert DM, Blanchard JW, Knox BL. Ensuring appropriate expert testimony for cases involving the "shaken baby." JAMA 2012;308(1):39-40.

[5] Niederkrotenthaler T, Xu L, Parks SE, Sugerman DE. Descriptive factors of abusive head trauma in young children—United States, 2000–2009. Child Abuse Negl 2013;37(7):446-55.

[6] Keenan HT, Runyan DK, Marshall SW, Nocera MA, Merten DF, Sinal SH. A population-based study of inflicted traumatic brain injury in young children. JAMA 2003;290(5):621-6.
[7] Barr RG, Trent RB, Cross J. Age-related incidence curve of hospitalized shaken baby syndrome cases: convergent evidence for crying as a trigger to shaking. Child Abuse Negl 2006;30(1):7-16.
[8] Caffey J. On the theory and practice of shaking infants: Its potential residual effects of permanent brain damage and mental retardation. Am J Dis Child 1972;124(2):161-9.
[9] Byard RW. "Shaken baby syndrome" and forensic pathology: An uneasy interface. Forens Sci Med Pathol 2014;10(239):e41.
[10] American Academy of Pediatrics Committee on Child Abuse and Neglect. Shaken baby syndrome: rotational cranial injuries—Technical report. Pediatrics 2001;108:206-10.
[11] Minns RA, Busuttil A. Patterns of presentation of the shaken baby syndrome: Four types of inflicted brain injury predominate. BMJ 2004;328(7442):766.
[12] Lazoritz S, Bier A. Historical perspectives. In: Lazoritz S, Palusci VJ, eds. The Shaken Baby Syndrome: A multidisciplinary approach. Binghamton, NY: Haworth Maltreatment and Trauma Press/Haworth Press, 2001:9-18.
[13] Caffey J. The parent-infant traumatic stress syndrome (Caffey-Kempe syndrome). Am J Roent Radiol Ther Nucl Med 1972;114(2):218-29.
[14] Reece RM, Nicholson CE, eds. Inflicted childhood neurotrauma. Elk Grove Village, IL: American Academy of Pediatrics, 2003.
[15] Christian CW, Block R. Abusive head trauma in infants and children. Pediatrics 2009;123(5):1409-11.
[16] Jenny C, Hymel KP, Ritzen A, Reinert SE, Hay TC. Analysis of missed cases of abusive head trauma. JAMA 1999;281(7):621-6.
[17] Wood JN, French B, Letson MM, Makoroff KL, Feldman KW, Fabio A, Berger R. Association of pediatric abusive head trauma rates with macroeconomic indicators. Acad Pediatr 2016;16(3):224-32.
[18] Miller TR, Steinbeigle R, Lawrence BA, Peterson C, Florence C, Barr M, Barr RG. Lifetime cost of abusive head trauma at ages 0–4, USA. Prev Sci 2018;19(6):695-704.
[19] Peterson C, Xu L, Florence C, Parks SE. Annual cost of U.S. hospital visits for pediatric abusive head trauma. Child Maltreat 2015;20(3):162-9.
[20] Scribano PV, Makoroff KL, Feldman KW, Berger RP. Association of perpetrator relationship to abusive head trauma clinical outcomes. Child Abuse Negl 2013;37(10):771-7.
[21] Esernio-Jenssen D, Tai J, Kodsi S. Abusive head trauma in children: A comparison of male and female perpetrators. Pediatr 2011;127(4):649-57.

[22] Ricci L, Giantris A, Merriam P, Hodge S, Doyle T. Abusive head trauma in Maine infants: Medical, child protective, and law enforcement analysis. Child Abuse Negl 2003;27(3):271-83.

[23] Adamsbaum C, Grabar S, Mejean N, Rey-Salmon C. Abusive head trauma: Judicial admissions highlight violent and repetitive trauma. Pediatrics 2010;126(3):546-55.

[24] Biron D, Shelton D. Perpetrator accounts in infant abusive head trauma brought about by a shaking event. Child Abuse Negl 2005;29(12):1347-58.

[25] Spivack BS. Biomechanics of abusive head trauma. J Aggress Maltreat Trauma 2001;5(1):55-78.

[26] Holbourn AHS. Mechanics of head injuries. Lancet 1943;242(6267):438-41.

[27] Ommaya AK, Faas F, Yarnell P. Whiplash injury and brain damage: An experimental study. JAMA 1968;204(4):285-9.

[28] Gennarelli TA, Thibault LE, Adams JH, Graham DI, Thompson CJ, Marcincin RP. Diffuse axonal injury and traumatic coma in the primate. Ann Neurol 1982;12(6):564-74.

[29] Imagawa KK, Hamilton A, Ceschin R, Tokar E, Pham P, Bluml S, Wisnowski J, Panigrahyet A. Characterization of microstructural injury: A novel approach in infant abusive head trauma—Initial experience. J Neurotrauma 2014;31(19):1632-8.

[30] Narang S, Clarke J. Abusive head trauma: Past, present, and future. J Child Neurol 2014;29(12):1747-56.

[31] Lind K, Toure H, Brugel D, Meyer P, Laurent-Vannier A, Chevignard M. Extended follow-up of neurological, cognitive, behavioral and academic outcomes after severe abusive head trauma. Child Abuse Negl 2016;51:358-67.

[32] Piteau SJ, Ward MK, Barrowman NJ, Plint AC. Clinical and radiographic characteristics associated with abusive and nonabusive head trauma: A systematic review. Pediatr 2012;30(2):315-23.

[33] Shein SL, Bell MJ, Kochanek PM, Tyler-Kabara EC, Wisniewski SR, Feldman K, Berger RP. Risk factors for mortality in children with abusive head trauma. J Pediatr 2012;161(4):716-22.

[34] Agrawal S, Peters MJ, Adams GG, Pierce CM. Prevalence of retinal hemorrhages in critically ill children. Pediatrics 2012;129(6):e1388-96.

[35] Coats B, Binenbaum G, Peiffer RL, Forbes BJ, Margulies SS. Ocular hemorrhages in neonatal porcine eyes from single, rapid rotational events. Invest Ophthal Visual Sci 2010;51(9):4792-7.

[36] Levin AV, Luyet FM, Knox BL. Ophthalmologic concerns in abusive head trauma. J Fam Violence 2016;31(7):797-804.

[37] Maguire SA, Watts PO, Shaw AD, Holden S, Taylor RH, Watkins WJ, Kemp AM. Retinal haemorrhages and related findings in abusive and non-abusive head trauma: A systematic review. Eye (Lond) 2013;27(1):28-36.

[38] Bhardwaj G, Chowdhury V, Jacobs MB, Moran KT, Martin FJ, Coroneo MT. A systematic review of the diagnostic accuracy of ocular signs in pediatric abusive head trauma. Ophthal 2010;117(5):983-92.

[39] Greeley CS. Abusive head trauma: A review of the evidence base. AJR 2015;204:967-73.

[40] Findley K, Barnes P, Moran D, Sperling C. Symposium examining Shaken Baby Syndrome convictions in light of new medical scientific research. Okla City UL Rev 2012;37:219-23.

[41] Tuerkheimer D. The next innocence project: shaken baby syndrome and the criminal courts. Wash UL Rev 2009;87(1):1-58.

[42] Henneberg M L. Admissibility frameworks and scientific evidence: controversies in relation to shaken baby syndrome/abusive head trauma. Br J Am Legal Stud 2015;4:555-83.

[43] Swedish Agency for Health Technology Assessment and Assessment of Social Services (SBU). Traumatic shaking: the role of the triad in medical investigations of suspected traumatic shaking - a systematic review. SBU assessment - report 255E. Stockhom, Sweden: SBU, 2016.

[44] Slovis TL, Strouse PJ, Coley BD, Rigsby CK. The creation of non-disease: an assault on the diagnosis of child abuse. Pediatr Radiol 2012;42:903-5.

[45] Narang S. A Daubert analysis of abusive head trauma/shaken baby syndrome. Hous J Health L Pol 2011;11:505-633.

[46] Narang SK, Melville JD, Greeley CS, Anderst JD, Carpenter SL, Spivack B. A Daubert analysis of abusive head trauma/shaken baby syndrome- Part II: An examination of the differential diagnosis. Hous J Health L Pol 2013;13:203-227.

[47] Narang SK, Greeley CS. Lynøe et al- #theRestoftheStory. Acta Pediatr 2017;106:1047-9.

[48] Debelle GD, Maguire S, Watts P, Hernandez RN, Kemp AM, on behalf of the Child Protection Standing Committee, Royal College of Paediatrics and Child Health. Abusive head trauma and the triad: A critique on behalf of the RCPCH of "Traumatic shaking: the role of the triad in medical investigations of suspected traumatic shaking.' Arch Dis Child 2018; 103(6):606-10.

[49] Gabaeff SC. Exploring the controversy in child abuse pediatrics and false accusations of abuse. Legal Medicine 2016;18,90-7.

[50] Krous HF, Byard RW. Controversies in pediatric forensic pathology. Forens Sci Med Pathol 2005;1(1), 9-18.

[51] Bazelon E. Shaken-baby syndrome faces new questions in court. New York Times Magazine 2011 Feb 06:30.

[52] Geddes JF, Plunkett J. The evidence base for shaken baby syndrome: Authors' reply. BMJ 2004;328(7451):1316-7.

[53] Geddes JF, Whitwell HL, Graham DI. Traumatic axonal injury: practical issues for diagnosis in medicolegal cases. Neuropathol Appl Neurobiol 2000;26(2):105-16.

[54] Geddes JF, Tasker RC, Hackshaw AK, Nickols CD, Adams GGW, Whitwell HL, et al. Dural haemorrhage in non-traumatic infant deaths: does it explain the bleeding in 'shaken baby syndrome'? Neuropathol Appl Neurobiol 2003;29(1):14-22.

[55] Choudhary AK, Servaes S, Slovis TL, Palusci VJ, Hedlund GL, Narang SK, et al. Consensus statement on abusive head trauma in infants and young children. Pediatr Rad 2018;48(8):1048-65.

[56] Stern P, Palusci VJ, Vandervort F, Hughes RC, Parrish R and the Abusive Head Trauma Committee. Promoting justice for victims of abusive head trauma: Information and strategy for effective courtroom presentation. Columbus, OH: APSAC Center for Child Policy, 2019. URL: http://www.centerforchildpolicy.org/assets/PromotingJusticeAHT.pdf.

[57] Edwards GA. Mimics of child abuse: Can choking explain abusive head trauma? J Forens Leg Med 2015;35:33-7.

[58] Jenny C. Alternate theories of causation in abusive head trauma: What the science tells us. Pediatr Radiol 2014;44(Suppl 4):S543-7.

[59] Hymel KP, Armijo-Garcia V, Foster R, Frazier TN, Stoiko M, Christie LM, Harper NS, Weeks K, Carroll CC, Hyden P, Sirotnak A, Truemper E, Ornstein AE, Wang M. Validation of a clinical prediction rule for pediatric abusive head trauma. Pediatrics 2014;134(6):e1537-48.

[60] Geddes JF, Hackshaw AK, Vowles GH, Nickols CD, Whitwell HL. Neuropathology of inflicted head injury in children: I. Patterns of brain damage. Brain 2001;124(7):1290-8.

[61] Narang SK, Estrada C, Greenberg S, Lindberg D. Acceptance of Shaken Baby Syndrome and Abusive Head Trauma as medical diagnoses. J Pediatr 2016;177:273-8.

[62] Strouse PJ. Child abuse: We have problems. Pediatr Radiol 2016 May;46(5):587-90.

[63] Christian CW, Committee on Child Abuse and Neglect, Section on Child Abuse and Neglect. Understanding abusive head trauma in infants and children: Answers from America's pediatricians. Elk Grove Village, IL: American Academy of Pediatrics, 2015. URL: https://www.aap.org/en-us/Documents/cocan_understanding_aht_in_infants_children.pdf.

[64] Barnes PD, Galaznik J, Gardner H, Shuman M. Infant acute life-threatening event--dysphagic choking versus nonaccidental injury. Semin Pediatr Neurol 2010;17:7-11.

[65] Lindberg DM, Dubowitz H, Alexander RC, Reece RM. The "new science" of abusive head trauma. Int J Child Maltreat Res Pol Pract 2019;2(1-2):1–16.

[66] Rao P, Carty H, Pierce A. The acute reversal sign: Comparison of medical and non-accidental injury patients. Clin Radiol 1999;54:495-501.

[67] Curcoy AI, Trenchs V, Morales M, Serra A, Pou J. Retinal hemorrhages and apparent life-threatening events. Pediatr Emerg Care 2010;26:118-20.

[68] Tucker J, Choudhary AK, Piatt J. Macrocephaly in infancy: Benign enlargement of the subarachnoid spaces and subdural collections. J Neurosurg Pediatr 2016;18:16-20.

[69] Lopes NRL, Eisenstein E, Williams LCA. Abusive head trauma in children: A literature review. J Pediatr (Rio J) 2013;89(5):426-33.

[70] Tanaka M, Jamieson E, Wathen N, MacMillan HL. Methodological standards for randomized controlled trials of interventions for preventing recurrence of child physical abuse and neglect. Child Abuse Rev 2010;19:21-38.

[71] Letson MM, Cooper JN, Deans KJ, Scribano PV, Makoroff KL, Feldman KW, Berger RP. Prior opportunities to identify abuse in children with abusive head trauma. Child Abuse Negl 2016;60:36-45.

[72] Sheets LK, Leach ME, Koszewski IJ, Lessmeier AM, Nugent M, Simpson P. Sentinel injuries in infants evaluated for child physical abuse. Pediatrics 2013;131(4):701-7.

[73] Bailhache M, Bénard A, Salmi L. Simulation of the impact of programs for prevention and screening of pediatric abusive head trauma. J Neurotrauma 2016;33(14):1397-1403.

[74] Hymel KP, Herman BE, Narang SK, Graf JM, Frazier TN, Stoiko M, Christie LM, Harper NS, Carroll CL, Boos SC, Dias M, Pullin DA, Wang M; Pediatric Brain Injury Research Network (PediBIRN) Investigators. Potential impact of a validated screening tool for pediatric abusive head trauma. J Pediatr 2015;167(6):1375-81.

[75] Cowley LE, Morris CB, Maguire SA, Farewell DM, Kemp AM. Validation of a prediction tool for abusive head trauma. Pediatrics 2015;136(2):291-8.

[76] Simonnet H, Laurent-Vannier A, Yuan W, Hully M, Valimahomed S, Bourennane M, Chevignard M. Parents' behavior in response to infant crying: Abusive head trauma education. Child Abuse Negl 2014;38(12):1914-22.

[77] Altman, RL, Canter J, Patrick PA, Daley N, Butt NK, Brand DA. Parent education by maternity nurses and prevention of abusive head trauma. Pediatrics 2011;128(5):e1164-74.

[78] Taşar MA, Bilge Y D, Şahin F, Çamurdan A, Beyazova U, Polat S, İlhan MN. Shaken baby syndrome prevention programme: A pilot study in turkey. Child Abuse Rev 2015;24(2):120-8.

[79] Barr RG. Preventing abusive head trauma resulting from a failure of normal interaction between infants and their caregivers. PNAS 2015;109(Suppl 2):17294-301.

[80] Barr RG, Barr M, Fujiwara T, Conway J, Catherine N, Brant R. Do educational materials change knowledge and behaviour about crying and shaken baby syndrome? A randomized controlled trial. Can Med Assoc J 2009;180(7):727-33.

[81] Fujiwara T, Yamada F, Okuyama M, Kamimaki I, Shikoro N, Barr RG. Effectiveness of educational materials designed to change knowledge and behavior about crying and shaken baby syndrome: A replication of a randomized controlled trial in Japan. Child Abuse Negl 2012;36(9):613-20.

[82] Barr RG, Barr M, Rajabali F, Humphreys C, Pike I, Brant R, Hlady J, Colbourne M, Fujiwara T, Singhal A. Eight-year outcome of implementation of abusive head trauma prevention. Child Abuse Negl 2018;84:106-14.

[83] Reese LS, Heiden EO, Kim KQ, Yang J. Evaluation of period of PURPLE Crying, an abusive head trauma prevention program. J Obstet Gynecol Neonat Nurs 2014;43(6): 752-61.

[84] Dias MS, Smith K, deGuehery K, Mazur P, Li V, Schaffer ML. Preventing abusive head trauma among infants and young children: A hospital based, parent education program. Pediatr 2005;115(4):470-7.

[85] Kelly P, Wilson K, Mowjood A, Freidman J, Reed P. Trialing a shaken baby syndrome prevention program in the Auckland District Health Board. NZ Med J 2016;129(1430):39-50.

[86] Morrill AC, McElaney L, Peixotto B, VanVleet M, Sege R. Evaluation of All Babies Cry, a second generation universal abusive head trauma prevention program. J Commun Psychol 2015;43(3):296-314.

[87] Dubowitz H. Feigelman S, Lane W, Kim J. Pediatric primary care to help prevent child maltreatment: The safe environment for every kid (SEEK) model. Pediatrics 2009;123(3):858-64.

[88] Dubowitz H. The safe environment for every kid (SEEK) model: Helping promote children's health, development, and safety: SEEK offers a practical model for enhancing pediatric primary care. Child Abuse Negl 2014;38(11):1725-33.

[89] Donelan-McCall N, Eckenrode J, Olds DL. Home visiting for the prevention of child maltreatment: lessons learned during the past 20 years. Pediatr Clin North Am 2009;56(2):389-403.

[90] Duggan AK, McFarlane EC, Fuddy L, Burrell LD, Higman S, Windham A, Sia C. Randomized trial of a statewide home visiting program: Impact in preventing child abuse and neglect. Child Abuse Negl 2004;28(6):597-622.

[91] McDonell JR, Ben-Arieh A, Melton GB. Strong communities for children: Results of a multi-year community-based initiative to protect children from harm. Child Abuse Negl 2015;41:79-96.

[92] Kimbrough-Melton RJ, Melton GB. 'Someone will notice, and someone will care': How to build strong communities for children. Child Abuse Negl 2015;41:67-78.

[93] Shanahan M, Fleming P, Nocera M, Sullivan K, Murphy R, Zolotor A. Process evaluation of a statewide abusive head trauma prevention program. Eval Progran Plann 2014;4:718-25.

[94] Hughes KN, Roygardner D, Palusci VJ. A structured review of the literature on abusive head trauma prevention. Child Abuse Rev 2020;29(3):in press.

[95] Roygardner D, Palusci VJ, Hughes KN. Advancing prevention zones: Implementing community-based strategies to prevent child maltreatment and promote healthy families. Int J Child Maltreat Res Pol Pract Online 2018 Nov 21. doi.10.1007/s42448-019-00039-0.

In: Building Children and Youth for the Future ISBN: 978-1-53618-806-6
Editors: Joav Merrick et al.

Chapter 4

THE IMPACT OF CONNECTEDNESS ON HARM REDUCTION IN CHILDREN AND ADOLESCENTS

Stephanie Stockburger*, MD, FAAP
Department of Pediatrics, Division of Adolescent Medicine,
University of Kentucky, Lexington, Kentucky,
United States of America

ABSTRACT

Adolescence is known to be a potentially turbulent time of physical, intellectual, personality, and social development. Adolescents may engage in high risk activities such as substance use, unprotected sex, and behaviors that contribute to unintentional injuries and violence. Adults can support adolescents and help curb risky behaviors. Multiple studies show that when adolescents feel connected to an adult at home, at school, or an adult mentor, adolescents are less likely to engage in risky behaviors.

* *Correspondence:* Stephanie Stockburger, MD, Associate Professor of Pediatrics, Department of Pediatrics, Division of Adolescent Medicine, 740 S Limestone, Lexington, KY 40536-0284, United States. Email: Sjstoc2@uky.edu.

INTRODUCTION

Adolescence is known to be a potentially turbulent time of physical, intellectual, personality, and social development. Adolescents are at increased risk of engaging in high risk behaviors such as substance use, sexual behaviors related to unintended pregnancy and sexually transmitted diseases including HIV, and behaviors that contribute to unintentional injuries and violence.

The Youth Risk Behavior Surveillance System (1) in the United States monitors health-risk behaviors that contribute to the leading causes of death and disability among youth and adults. The YRBSS population consists of representative samples of students typically in grades 9-12. The 2017 survey found that 14% of high school students had ever used illicit drugs, 14% had ever misused prescription opioids, and 1.5% had ever injected illegal drugs (1). Regarding sexual behavior, 39.5% had ever had sex, 53.8% had used a condom during last sexual intercourse, 29.4% used effective birth control, and 8.8% used a condom and effective hormonal birth control (1). Violent behaviors were also surveyed. The 2017 survey found that 6% of high school students were threatened or injured with a weapon at school, 6.7% did not go to school because of safety concerns, 14.9% were electronically bullied, and 19% were bullied at school (1). In addition, violent dating and sexual behaviors were surveyed. The survey found that 7.4% reported that they were forced to have sex, 8% experienced physical dating violence, and 6.9% experienced sexual dating violence (1). Regarding mental health and suicide variables, the survey found that 31.3% had experienced persistent feelings of sadness or hopelessness, 17.2% seriously considered attempting suicide, 13.6% had a suicide plan, 7.4% had attempted suicide, and 2.4% were injured in a suicide attempt (1).

Why do teens engage in high risk behaviors? The answer is that it's normal for teens to want to try new experiences. Teens need to explore their own limits and abilities as well as boundaries that are set. They also need to express themselves as individuals. All of this exploring and boundary pushing is part of their path to becoming independent young adults with their own identities (2). Adolescent brains are going through profound changes (2). Structural changes are occurring during brain development. Main changes are occurring in the pre-frontal cortex, amygdala, nucleus accumbens, and cerebellum (2). The pre-frontal cortex controls executive functions and is the last area of the brain to fully develop (3). Executive functions are the higher-level cognitive skills that control and coordinate cognitive abilities and behaviors (3). Organization and regulation are executive functions (3). Organization includes attention, planning, sequencing, problem-solving, working memory, cognitive flexibility, abstract thinking, rule acquisition, and selecting relevant sensory information (3). Regulation includes initiation of action, self-control, emotional regulation, monitoring internal and external stimuli, initiating and inhibiting context-specific behavior, moral reasoning, and decision making (3). The amygdala of the brain regulates emotion and associated memory. The nucleus accumbens is the center for motivation, reward, and punishment. The cerebellum controls co-ordination and balance. All of these parts of the brain are maturing during adolescence.

As the pre-frontal cortex of the brain is not mature during adolescence, adolescents may have difficulty truly understanding the consequences of their actions and regulating their behavior. As the amygdala and nucleus accumbens are still maturing, adolescents may seek stimulating and exciting experiences and have more tumultuous emotional experiences. Dr. Ron Dahl, a psychologist at the University of Pittsburgh stated "teens are like high-powered cars without skilled drivers" (2).

Although we may now have a better understanding of why teens are more prone to risky behaviors, further framing the behaviors as part of the natural development of adolescents can be helpful. It is important to note that for adolescents, as for adults, all behaviors serve a purpose. In other words, behaviors are situational expressions of maturational events (2). We tend to objectify the behaviors, as in this paper, and label them as "risk taking" or "health compromising" (2). However, adolescents may feel that their behaviors are part of a solution. For example, if a teen feels like they don't fit in with their peers and they see their peers using marijuana, they may try marijuana to fit in. For this teen, using marijuana is a solution to the problem of feeling like they don't fit in. Just like adults, teens may also use substances (or have other "risky" behaviors) for stress relief or as a coping mechanism. An adult may turn to a cigarette to cope with stress. An adolescent may do the same. It can be helpful to reframe adolescent behaviors. We may be tempted to respond to an adolescent's behavior with "what's wrong with you?" Instead, we could (and should) reframe this with "what's going on with you?"

CONNECTEDNESS TO FAMILY, SCHOOL, AND MENTORS

Now that we have a better understanding of what is going on with an adolescent's development and brain maturation, the question becomes: how can we decrease an adolescent's risk of adverse health consequences? We can decrease adolescent's risk of adverse health consequences by increasing an adolescent's sense of connectedness especially to their family or school. Connectedness is an important protective factor for youth. Connectedness refers to a sense of being cared for, supported, and belonging. It can be centered on feeling connected to school, family (i.e., parents and caregivers) or other important people and organizations. Youth who feel connected at school and at home are less likely to experience negative health outcomes related to sexual risk, substance use, violence, and mental health (4).

An article from the journal of Pediatrics titled "Adolescent connectedness and adult health outcomes" found that school connectedness in adolescence had protective associations in adulthood (5). The authors found that school connectedness reduced emotional distress and odds of suicidal ideation (5). They also found reduced physical violence victimization and perpetration in adolescents who felt connected at school (5). In addition, school connectedness had protective associations regarding multiple sex partners, sexually transmitted infection (STI) diagnosis, prescription drug misuse, and other illicit drug use (5). The same article noted that family connectedness also had multiple protective effects (5). Family connectedness has protective effects for emotional distress, all violence indicators including intimate sex partner violence, multiple sex partners, STI diagnosis, and substance use indicators (5). The article concluded that "family and school connectedness may have long-lasting protective effects across health outcomes related to mental health, violence, sexual behavior and substance use" (5).

A study of urban, ethnically diverse students in a school-based mentoring program found that a high quality youth mentor relationship was significantly associated with positive social, academic, and health-related behaviors (6). The same authors also found that parent-youth connectedness in a statewide sample of high school students who reported homelessness in the past year concluded that all measures of parent connectedness were significantly associated with lower sexual risk levels (6).

School connectedness is the belief held by students that adults and peers care about their learning as well as about them as individuals (7). Students are more likely to succeed academically and engage in healthy behaviors when they feel connected to their school (8). Young people who feel connected to their school are less likely to engage in risky behaviors including early sexual initiation, substance use, violence, and gang involvement (8). Academically, students who feel connected to their school are more likely to have better academic achievement (8). They are more likely to have higher grades, higher test scores, better attendance, and stay in school longer (8).

School connectedness has also been found to decrease suicidal thoughts and attempts. A meta-analysis evaluated school connectedness and suicidal thoughts and attempts. The authors found that students reporting a connection to their schools are significantly less likely to report having suicidal thoughts or report making a suicide attempt (9).

To increase school connectedness, the Centers for Disease Control and Prevention (CDC) recommends that schools use several strategies (10). Schools can create decision-making processes that promote family, community, and student engagement 10). These decision-making processes should facilitate academic achievement and staff empowerment (10). Schools can also providc opportunitics for families to be actively involved in their child's academic and school life (10). In addition, schools can provide students with the necessary academic, social, and emotional skills to be engaged in school (10). School districts and administrators can support teachers in using effective classroom management and teaching methods which promote a positive learning environment (10). Schools can provide professional development and support for teachers and school staff to help them meet the diverse cognitive, emotional, and social needs of their students (10). Finally, schools can create trusting and caring relationships that promote open communication between students, staff, teachers, and administration (10).

Families and caregivers can take action to promote school connectedness with their children and adolescents. They can communicate openly and honestly, including about their values (11). Families and caregivers can supervise their adolescent to promote healthy decision-making (11). They can become engaged in school activities and participate in volunteer activities at the school (11). They may offer to help their child or adolescent with homework, if needed (11). Spending time with the child or adolescent enjoying shared activities helps them feel more engaged (11). Families and caregivers can also communicate regularly with teachers and administrators (11). If families and caregivers take steps to engage and connect themselves to the school community, children and adolescents will likely also feel more connected to the school.

ONLINE CONNECTEDNESS

Most teens in the United States are not only connected with school, peers, and families, but also with the global online community. This presents different benefits, as well as challenges, when compared with previous generations of adolescents. Most teens feel that social media has a positive effect on how they feel about themselves. According to an article from the Common Sense Media website, 25% of teens say social media makes them feel less lonely, 8% say it makes them feel better about themselves, and 16% say it makes them feel less depressed (12). Fewer teens feel the opposite. Three percent of teens report that social media makes them feel lonelier, 4% report they feel worse about themselves, and 3% report they feel more depressed when using social media (12). Fewer teens are reporting being cyberbullied. In a 2019 report, only 13% of teens reported ever being cyberbullied (12). However, almost two-thirds of teens report they often or sometimes come across racist, sexist, homophobic, or religious-based hate content while using social media (12).

Parents and guardians can guide adolescents toward healthier social media use. Adolescents may have difficulty regulating their own screen time. Parents and caregivers can set limits on screen time and have screen-free time periods or "zones" including homework time, bedtime, and family meal time (12). Caregivers can also check in frequently about adolescents social media use. If there is an individual that is bringing the teen down, caregivers can encourage the adolescent to block the individual, report, or unfriend that person (12).

IMPROVING FAMILY CONNECTEDNESS

Families can take steps to improve connectedness, improve effectiveness of discipline, and enforce rules regarding safety. Most importantly, parents and guardians should take time to actively listen to their children and adolescents. To actively listen, parents and guardians should stop what they are doing and give the child or adolescent their full attention, and allow the child to talk without interrupting (13). Actively listening builds relationships and improves connectedness. Adolescents who feel more connected to their caregiver(s) are more likely to have fewer discipline problems. Caregivers can work on choosing their battles instead of fighting or having conflict over small things (13). By doing this, caregivers can save their energy for larger battles, especially issues that involve safety (13). Additionally important for caregivers is to be on the same page as other caregivers. This helps provide a united front, especially for major issues, like rules related to safety (13). Another strategy is to set limits and agree on them with the adolescent (13). Discussing consequences ahead of time can help the adolescent make informed choices about their behavior. Also, it may be helpful to be willing to discuss and adjust rules as teens show responsibility is important (13).

In addition, studies show that having dinner together as a family may decrease risky behaviors and foster togetherness (14). In families who have infrequent family dinners, less than three times per week, adolescents were found to be twice as likely to have used tobacco, almost twice as likely to have used alcohol, and are 1 ½ times likelier to have used marijuana (14). Families that have family dinners together at least three times a week are more likely to be more connected.

> It is easier to build a strong child than to repair a broken man
> Frederick Douglass

Improving Family Connectedness: The Danish Way

In their book called "The Danish way of parenting" Jessica Alexander and Iben Sandahl use the acronym PARENT to describe how Danes parent their children (15). Denmark has consistently been voted one of the happiest countries in the world for over 40 years. One of the authors, Jessica Alexander, is an American who is married to a Dane (15). She noticed that the way the Danes parent their children is different than the American way (15). In the book, the authors urge readers to remove their "cultural glasses" for a moment and try on a "Danish way" of seeing things (15). The acronym PARENT that is used stands for play, authenticity, reframing, empathy, no ultimatums, togetherness and hygge (15). The term "default settings" is added after the acronym as this is how we tend to parent when we are stressed and overwhelmed (15).

P is for Play

In the acronym, PARENT, the "p" stands for play (15). The authors discuss that play is a very important part of a child's development and that children need time to play freely (15). Play helps children develop a sense of self that shapes the foundation for whole and happy children (15). Play teaches children to be less anxious and more resilient (15). When children play, that have the experience of succeeding with something new (16). When children are allowed to experiment freely, the authors state that endorphins are released in the reward system of the child's brain which leads to feelings of happiness and satisfaction (16). Play also improves social skills (16). Being given the space to play freely makes the child feel like they are in control of their lives which leads to greater autonomy and self-control (15).

Family play is also important for children and healthy families (16). As family play does not seem to be a huge part of the American culture, this may seem different and challenging especially at first. Instead of thinking about play as something that happens when there is nothing else going on, try to make it a priority. In order for this to happen, many of us may need to challenge our mindset and remind ourselves that play is not lazy, it has profound benefits (16). A good way to add family play is to start with physical play, even for 10-15 minutes after work (16). In addition to physical play, think about creative, emotional, social, digital, and cognitive play (16). Play can be silly. Chores can be gamified (6). Try not to worry about "making a mess" and instead "think creativity" (16). Messes can be cleaned up, but the benefits of free and creative play will be reaped for years (16)! Family play helps the family connect and reap the benefits of connectedness.

A IS FOR AUTHENTICITY

In the book "A Danish way of parenting" it is mentioned that while Americans tend to watch movies with happy endings, Danish moves are typically not this way (15). Danes watch movies with dreary or sad endings. The authors state that Danes believe that tragedies and upsetting events are important to talk about too (15). In Denmark, there is more of an emphasis on understanding one's own emotions and allowing children to see that a range of emotions is normal (16). What is important is to learn how to deal with these emotions (15). When the obstacle has passed, parents can have a discussion with their children about how they were feeling and what was helpful for them (15). Being authentic is an important tool to help families connect.

R IS FOR REFRAMING

In the book, the authors discuss that reframing is crucial to resilience (15). All situations can be reframed in a more positive way (15). For example, in America, two year old behavior is commonly referred to as the "terrible two's." In Denmark, this age is called the "boundary pushing" age. Reframing a toddler's behavior changes it from "terrible" to being something that is normal for their developmental age (15). There are many examples of reframing. In the book, an example is a soccer game being rained out but instead the family has time for a monopoly tournament. Parents need to lead this positive trend in reframing their own situations. Children will learn this skill from their parents! Again, this is a critical skill for building resilience (15)!

> The best and most beautiful things in the world cannot be seen, they must be touched with the heart
>
> Helen Keller (16)

E IS FOR EMPATHY

Empathy is the ability to recognize and feel the feelings of others (15). Since the 1980s and 1990s, empathy in college students has dropped by 50% (15). Students are scoring increasingly higher in narcissism (15). In America, individualism is highly valued as is being "the best" and standing out at something (15). American culture is definitely more focused on "I" than "we." However, we are actually wired to be closer to others (15).

Babies will try to soothe other babies and toddlers will pick up something an adult accidentally drops (15). Humans have survived over the years because we have collaborated, not because we have gone out on our own (15). We may actually get more pleasure from making others happy than making ourselves happy (15). It is important to approach others, and our children, with understanding. If our child is unusually fussy or upset, think about whether they could be tired or hungry (15). Be mindful of how you talk about other children as well as other adults. Remember to have compassion for others and avoid labeling others negatively, especially in front of your child (15). Instead, have empathy and teach your children to have empathy (15). For example, "Johnny may have acted out on the school bus today, but maybe he didn't get enough sleep last night or maybe he was hungry." We are able to connect more closely to others if we allow ourselves to have empathy.

N IS FOR NO ULTIMATUMS

An ultimatum is stating "if you do (or don't do) this, then this will happen." Ultimatums put parents in a position where there has to be a winner and a loser (15). It is a power struggle (15). It does not offer a win/win solution (15). Instead, govern with respect. When parents resort to screaming, spanking, or shaming to get results, children lose respect for their parents and may learn that screaming, hitting, and saying mean worse is how to get someone to do something you want them today (15). Children mirror their parents. Remember that good begets good, bad begets bad, out of control begets out of control, and calm begets calm (15). Parents lose closeness by governing with threats and fear (15). If parents genuinely see their children as intrinsically good and base their reactions to them on that knowledge, they tend to be more respectful and empathetic (15). Try to understand why children are having certain behaviors (book). That being said, children do need firm rules and boundaries (15). Help children understand why the rules and boundaries are there (15).

T IS FOR TOGETHERNESS

In Denmark, there is something called "hygge" which means "to be cozy" (15). Families set aside time to just be together and "cozy around." They often light candles and have tea and cake (15). They all pitch in so there is not one or two people being left with all of the work (15). They use this time to be fully present with each other and value the time together with children or family (15). The television and electronic devices are off (15). Drama is "left" at the door (15). People do not gossip or say mean things about each other. In Denmark, families may get together and do this for days (15). Perhaps this is missing in America. There is much evidence that a strong support system builds our immune system and helps us fight viruses, such as the common cold virus (15). In fact, if "we" is substituted for "I" in the word "illness" it becomes "wellness" (15). Improved physical and mental health may be benefits of togetherness time or "hygge." In America, is this way of being together is less common, families could start in a small way, spending 10 minutes of "togetherness" time to start. The authors state that it is okay for this time to have a time limit (16).

DEFAULT SETTINGS

Our default settings kick in when we are tired, stressed, or overwhelmed (15). Our default settings are rooted in how we were parented (15). If we think back to how we were parented, was it based on respect and empathy? Were there ultimatums, spanking, yelling, and power struggles? Or were we respected and listened to? If our default settings are falling short of being effective or positive, we should question, could another way be better (15)?

CONCLUSION

In conclusion, connectedness at school and at home has been shown to reduce a variety of health risk behaviors. Connectedness refers to a sense of being cared for, supported, and belonging. Youth who feel connected at school and home are less likely to experience negative health outcomes related to sexual risk, substance use, violence, and mental health. The common goal is to help young people navigate adolescence while building strengths and decreasing risky behaviors. Families, schools, and mentors can help youth feel more connected and reduce potential harmful behaviors.

REFERENCES

[1] CDC.gov [Internet]. Washington, D.C.: CDC releases 2017 Youth Risk Behavior Survey (YRBS) results: 2018 June 14 [cited 2020 Feb 8]. Centers for Disease Control and Prevention. URL: https://www.cdc.gov/nchhstp/dear_colleague/2018/dcl-061418-YRBS.html.

[2] Omar H. The teen brain [PowerPoint]. Lexington, KY: University of Kentucky, 2016.

[3] University of California San Francisco, San Francisco, CA: Executive functions, 2020. Weill Institute for Neurosciences: Memory and aging center. URL: https://memory.ucsf.edu/symptoms/executive-functions.

[4] CDC.gov [Internet]. Washington, D.C.: Adolescent connectedness; 2019 Aug 21. Centers for Disease Control and Prevention. URL: https://www.cdc.gov/healthy youth/protective/youth-connectedness-important-protective-factor-for-health-well-being.htm.

[5] Steiner RJ, Sheremenko G, Lesesne C, Dittus PJ, Dittus RE, Sieving RE, Ethier KA. Adolescent connectedness and adult health outcomes. Pediatrics 2019;144(1). URL: https://pediatrics.aappublications.org/content/144/1/e20183766.

[6] Sieving RE, McRee A, McMorris BJ, Shlafar RJ, Gower AL, Kapa HM, et al. Youth-adult connectedness: A key protective factor for adolescent health. Am J Prev Med 2017;52(3S3):S275-78.

[7] CDC.gov [Internet]. Washington, DC: Adolescent and school health: School connectedness; 2018 Aug 7. URL: https://www.cdc.gov/healthyyouth/protective/school_connectedness.htm.

[8] American Psychological Association. Washington, DC: School connectedness, 2020. URL: https://www.apa.org/pi/lgbt/programs/safe-supportive/school-connectedness.

[9] Marraccini ME, Brier ZM. School connectedness and suicidal thoughts and behaviors: a systematic meta-analysis. Sch Psychol Q 2017;32(1):5-21.

[10] CDC.gov [Internet]. Washington, DC: Fostering school connectedness: Information for school districts and school administrators, 2009. URL: https://www.cdc.gov/healthyyouth/protective/pdf/connectedness_administrators.pdf.

[11] CDC.gov [Internet]. Washington, DC: Fostering school connectedness: Information for parents and families 2019 Nov 21. URL: https://www.cdc.gov/healthyyouth/protective/factsheets/connectedness_parents.htm.

[12] Knorr C. Parenting, media, and everything in between: What teens really think about their social media lives. San Francisco, CA: Common Sense Media, 2018 Sept 8. URL: https://www.commonsensemedia.org/blog/what-teens-really-think-about-their-social-media-lives.

[13] Raisingchildren.net.au [Internet]. Teens: Communicating and relationships. Australia: Raising Children Network, 2006-2020. URL: https://raisingchildren.net.au/teens/communicating-relationships.

[14] Centeronaddiction.org [Internet]. The importance of family dinners VIII. New York: Center on Addiction, 2012. URL: https://www.centeronaddiction.org/addiction-research/reports/importance-of-family-dinners-2012.

[15] Alexander JJ, Sandahl ID. The Danish way of parenting: What the happiest people in the world know about raising confident, capable kids. New York: TarcherPerigee, 2016.

[16] Alexander JJ, Sandahl ID. What the happiest people in the world know about raising confident, capable kids. URL: http://thedanishway.com/.

In: Building Children and Youth for the Future ISBN: 978-1-53618-806-6
Editors: Joav Merrick et al.

Chapter 5

SUICIDE IN ADOLESCENTS: EXPLORING THE ROLE OF RELIGION

Minh Nguyen, DO, Maria Demma Cabral*, MD and Dilip R Patel, MD, MBA, MPH
Department of Medicine-Pediatrics and Department of Pediatric and Adolescent Medicine, Western Michigan University Homer Stryker MD School of Medicine, Kalamazoo, Michigan, United States of America

ABSTRACT

Suicide in most religious beliefs is forbidden. Some studies have implicated that affiliating with a religious or spiritual group can have a positive impact for an individual going through depression and suicide. However, in some studies, there had been concern that religion can be a risk factor. With the ever-changing religious face of the world, it is

* *Correspondence:* Maria Demma Cabral, MD, Assistant Professor, Department of Pediatric and Adolescent Medicine, Western Michigan University Homer Stryker MD School of Medicine, Kalamazoo, Michigan, United States.
Email: Mariademma.cabral@med.wmich.edu.

important to recognize its significance, or lack of, particularly in caring for depressed and suicidal youth.

INTRODUCTION

There are many definitions of religion, depending on a myriad of factors including cultures, social contexts, community settings, and others. In general, religion regards a commitment or devotion to religious faith or observance. It also features a personal set or institutional system of religious attitudes, beliefs and practices. Most importantly, it involves a relationship with God. Religion plays an integral part in people's lives, across geographical boundaries and age groups. This chapter will explore the role of religion in adolescence, particularly in the context of suicide, considering that adolescence is an essential phase of physical and psychologic growth.

A BRIEF LOOK INTO RELIGION

According to the "World Christian encyclopedia: A comparative survey of churches and religions in the modern world," 19 major religions share the Earth (1). A closer look shows these are further subdivided into 270 large religious groups with many smaller ones. A study from the Pew Research Center in 2017 showed that Christianity remains the world's largest religion, followed by Islam, Hinduism, Buddhism and Judaism (2). Moving onto the future, religious profile of the world will continue to change rapidly, driven by differences in fertility rates and the size of youth populations among the world's major religions. Islam is currently the fastest growing religion and by 2050, the projection is that there will be as many Muslims as Christians around the world (2).

It is vital to discuss spirituality in the context of religion. Religion and spirituality share many overlapping concepts and may be used interchangeably. Spirituality is defined as "sensitivity or attachment to religious values" (3). In the same study from the Pew Research Center, adults younger than age 40 are found to be less likely to identity with a religion, believe in God or engage in religious practices, especially in the United States and Canada. In fact, the rates of atheists, agnostics and unaffiliated is declining across the world, but increasing in the United States (3).

Gearing and Lizardi (4) and Gearing and Alonzo (5), performed a comprehensive review of literature from 1908 to 2017 on religion, focusing on Christianity, Hinduism, Islam and Judaism, and suicide. The fundamental notion is that religion provides protection against suicide, among those who are religiously committed, engaged in their religious community, and living in an area of high religiosity. At a closer look, the degree of protection from suicide varies widely across religions. Suicides rates are relatively higher in Christianity and Hinduism compared to Islam and Judaism, although there are several factors that should be considered (4, 5). In Christianity, particularly Catholics, suicide is in violation of the sixth commandment: "Thou shall not kill." It has been observed that rates of suicide decline come Christmas and surges come New Year (5). In Islam, it has been thought that there may be significant under-reporting of suicide due to strong social stigma and shame and that mental-related help could be scarce (5).

Religion in youth

Adolescence is the age group of focus in this chapter based on implications of suicide in a person's life. Numerous habits and coping skills that adults acquired overtime are initiated and learned during their adolescent years. In fact, under-addressed or unrecognized mental health challenges during adolescence can have a lifelong impact and result in early mortality by suicide. Suicide remains one of the leading causes of death in youth.

The American Academy of Child and Adolescent Psychiatry (6) and the Centers for Disease Control and Prevention (7) have listed factors in youth suicide. There are well known factors including depression, family history of suicide attempts, access of firearms for risk factors, and effective comprehensive clinical care, easy access to mental health services for protective factors. Notably, cultural and religious beliefs play a role in both categories (6, 7). For adolescents who may be struggling with their place in the world, it is important to explore how their religious belief may impact how strongly they feel about living. Rates of American youth identifying as non-affiliated to any religious group have been rising. Geographically, teens from the South were considered most religious (8).

There is ample data on the protective mechanism of religion. Yonker et al. (9) demonstrated in their study in that spirituality/religion had an overall protective effect on adolescents and emerging adults. Work from Svobo et al. (10) suggested that parental attitudes towards religion play a role in their child's risk for suicide. Similarly, in a paper published by Bullock et al. (11), if youth feel connected to a member of the religious community, they may be more likely to seek help and be referred for additional support from a mental health professional (11).

In contrast, religious practices in privacy, lack of spiritual conviction and faithful beliefs of God's anger, and punishment and doubt were negatively predictive of poorer mental health and suicide. One sample study found these individuals had increased likelihood of being hopeless and depressed, reporting less likely to attend and be active in church (12). Sexual minority youth may feel even less connected to a certain religion and hence their risk of depression and suicide may be heightened (13). In addition, rates of attempted suicide continue to increase among minority groups, yet it is unclear if the certain risk and protective factors are less or more pertinent to being at higher risk.

PROTECTIVE AND HARMFUL MECHANISMS OF RELIGION TOWARD SUICIDE

There are several postulated mechanisms of protection from religion against suicide including strongly condemning the act; providing a supportive community; decreasing aggressive behaviors and violence; disapproving substance use and smoking; and establishing a positive, optimistic perspective on life (4, 5). Based on a systematic review of the literature by Lawrence et al. (14), religious affiliation was shown to offer protection against suicide attempts, the severity of suicide attempts, and completed suicide. Religious service attendance is another component that demonstrated protective effect in the same study. It is important to point out that there is adequate evidence suggesting the effect of religious service attendance while adjusting for social support resulting from attending services as a possible confounder. The protective effect of religion may also be explained by providing skills to cope with and/or incentives to endure hardship or suicidal thoughts: promoting certain beliefs such as "moral and religious objections to suicide"; giving hope and reassurance of divine control (14).

However, religion may amplify suicide risk in certain individuals who experience 'negative religious coping,' which may involve deferring all responsibility to God, feeling abandoned by God, blaming God for difficulties, experiencing spiritual tension or doubt or guilt, or experiencing conflict and struggle with God. Religion may not be as protective against suicide for certain individuals that are less accepted by their own religious community, an example being those with mental illnesses. For a subset of individuals, increased religious activity such as praying more frequently may be a response to increased emotional distress, not necessarily a productive coping method (15).

PROPOSED GUIDELINES FOR SUICIDE RISK EVALUATION

Gearing and Lizardi (4) had proposed guidelines when assessing the at-risk individual taking into account one's 'spiritual competence.' One must determine significance of the person's religion to self and to others (i.e., family). It is necessary to understand if religion resonates with the person's identity. Asking the person if they know of the concept of suicide and how it is perceived in their religion. It helps recognize role of being religion in relation to stressful and difficult times. And lastly, how strong does the person feel connected and the extent of participation the person does in relation to affiliated religious beliefs.

There may be value in utilizing these steps particularly in youth who strongly identifies with the religion they affiliate with. Exploring the youth's beliefs can help dictate management that can target suicide behavior and be a useful tool in preventing unwarranted deaths.

Conclusion

In most studies, religion has been identified as a protective factor in suicide. But it has also been shown to be have a negative impact. Considering that the rates of depression and suicide in youth continue to rise at an alarming rate, it is imperative for the clinician to include questions about religious or spiritual beliefs routinely. Such promotes positive thoughts and behaviors in addressing suicidality. Studies looking at religion and its role in suicide especially the youth is limited, and more is needed to address the knowledge gap in this topic.

Acknowledgments

This chapter is an updated and revised version of an earlier publication: Cabral MD et al. Role of religion in adolescent suicide. In: Shatahmasebi S, Omar HA, eds. Suicide: A broader view. Cambridge: Cambridge Scholars Publishing, 2019 with permission.

References

[1] Barrett DB, Kurian GT, Johnson TM. World Christian Encyclopedia: The world segments: religions, peoples, languages, cities, topics. New York: Oxford University Press, 2001.

[2] Pew Research Center. The changing global religious landscape. 2017. URL: https://www.pewforum.org/2017/04/05/the-changing-global-religious-landscape/.

[3] Definition of spiritual. Merriam-Webster, Inc. URL: https://www.merriam-webster.com/dictionary/spiritual.

[4] Gearing RE, Lizardi D. Religion and suicide. J Relig Health 2009;48:332-42.

[5] Gearing RE, Alonzo D. Religion and suicide: New findings. J Relig Health 2018;57:2478-99.

[6] American Academy of Child and Adolescent Psychiatry. Suicide in children and teens. Facts for families. 2018. URL: https://www.aacap.org/AACAP/Families_and_Youth/Facts_for_Families/FFF-Guide/Teen-Suicide-010.aspx.

[7] Centers for Disease Control and Prevention. Suicide: Risk and protective factors. 2019. URL: https://www.cdc.gov/violenceprevention/suicide/riskprotectivefactors.html.

[8] King PE, Roeser RW. Religion and spirituality in adolescent development. In: Lerner RM, Steinberg L, eds. Handbook of adolescent psychology: Individual bases of adolescent development, 3rd edition. Hoboken, NJ: John Wiley Sons, 2009:435-78.

[9] Yonker J, Schnabelrauch C, DeHaan L. The relationship between spirituality and religiosity on psychological outcomes in adolescents and emerging adults: a meta-analytic review. J Adolescence 2012;35(2):299-314.

[10] Svobo C, Wickramaratne J, Reich L, Zhao R, Talati A, Gameroff M. Association of parent and offspring religiosity with offspring suicide ideation and attempts. JAMA Psychiatry 2018;75(10):1062-70.

[11] Bullock M, Nadeau L, Renaud J. Spirituality and religion in youth suicide attempters' trajectories of mental health service utilizations: the year before a suicide attempt. J. Can Acad Child Adolesc Psychiatry 2011;21(3)186-92.

[12] Molock SD, Puri R, Matlin S, Barksdale C. Relationship between religious coping and suicidal behaviors among African American adolescents. JBlack Psychol 2006;32(3)366–89.

[13] Gibbs J. Religious conflict, sexual identity, and suicidal behaviors among LGBT young adults. Arch Suicide Res 2015;194(4):472-88.

[14] Lawrence RE. Religion and suicide risk: a systematic review. Arch Suicide Res 2016;20:1-21.

[15] Regnerus M, Uecker J. Finding faith, losing faith: The prevalence and context of religious transformations during adolescence. Rev Religious Res 2006;47:217-37.

In: Building Children and Youth for the Future ISBN: 978-1-53618-806-6
Editors: Joav Merrick et al.

Chapter 6

ADVERSE CHILDHOOD EXPERIENCES AND SUBSTANCE USE DISORDER: EXPLORING CONNECTIONS AND TRAUMA INFORMED CARE

Madelyn J McDonald*[*]*, MPH
Center for Innovation in Population Health, College of Public Health,
University of Kentucky, Lexington, Kentucky,
United States of America

ABSTRACT

Adverse childhood experiences (ACEs) include abuse, neglect, and household dysfunction experienced between the ages of 0 and 17 years. These quantifiable experiences can be expressed as an ACE score of 1 to 10. Between 1995 and 1997, the Centers for Disease Control and Prevention (CDC) conducted a study examining the prevalence and

[*] *Correspondence:* Madelyn J McDonald, MPH, Policy Analyst, University of Kentucky, Center for Innovation in Population Health, 364 Healthy Kentucky Building, Lexington, KY 40506, United States. Email: madelyn.mcdonald@uky.edu.

effects of the 10 categories of ACEs, and found that ACEs are common yet commonly go unrecognized, and can lead to myriad health and social impacts later in life1. Among the most significant of these impacts is a 4- to 12-fold increase in risk for depression, suicide, and substance abuse1. Data has shown that trauma increases risk for addiction and substance use disorder (SUD), sometimes as a means of comfort or self-treatment2. Considering a trauma-informed care approach for those with SUD and other addiction disorders, particularly those with a history of ACEs, could change the treatment landscape and promote recovery.

INTRODUCTION

An adolescent seeks treatment at a substance use disorder (SUD) treatment clinic for intermittent heroin injection, but is turned away due to dropping out of treatment several times in the past. Although counselors at the clinic want the adolescent to achieve full recovery, they are discouraged by the patient's pattern of relapsing each time he seems to be on the path to recovery, and have developed the idea that he is simply not ready for treatment. However, although routine counseling is a mandatory component of treatment at this clinic, the patient has undisclosed trauma that had not come up in these sessions. Without addressing this underlying issue, recovery from SUD will be much more difficult for this patient (1, 2).

DEFINING ADVERSE CHILDHOOD EXPERIENCES

Adverse childhood experiences (ACEs) occur during young life (0-17 years of age), and include potentially traumatic events such as experiencing or witnessing violence or abuse. The 10 categories of ACEs can be broken down into three main themes:

- Childhood abuse: emotional, physical, or sexual
- Childhood neglect: emotional or physical

- Household dysfunction: witnessing domestic violence, substance abuse, mental illness, and parental incarceration, separation, or divorce

An ACE score can be calculated by asking questions such as "Between the ages of 1 and 17, did you experience . . . in your household?" and adding up the responses for an ACE score of 0 to 10.

According to the CDC, ACEs are common in the United States, with close to 61% of adults reporting at least one type of ACE, and about 1 in 6 reporting four or more types of ACEs (3). People of all backgrounds can experience ACEs, but they are most common among women and racial and ethnic minority groups (3).

ACEs have been linked to widespread health effects in adulthood including risky health behaviors, chronic health conditions, low life potential, and early death (3). Lasting impacts can include, but are not limited to, the following:

- Depression and anxiety
- Suicide
- PTSD
- Physical injury
- Unsafe sex
- Unintended pregnancy & pregnancy complications
- Diabetes
- Heart disease
- Cancer
- COPD
- Loss of educational and occupational opportunities
- Alcohol and drug abuse

Of particular significance is the increase in suicidal ideation – compared to those with no ACEs, those with four or more ACEs have shown a 4- to 12-fold increase in suicide attempts1. Additional research has shown that ACEs may be associated with increased suicide risk among US military veterans who also suffer from PTSD (4).

PREVENTING ADVERSE CHILDHOOD EXPERIENCES

ACEs can be prevented by strengthening economic support to families, promoting social norms that protect against violence and adversity, teaching skills to new parents, and early intervention (3). However, prevention of ACEs can be difficult, and these improvements to individual family life often require bigger, society-level changes to see meaningful impacts (1). Home visitation programs like HANDS, and interventions like the Positive Parenting Program, are examples of successful primary prevention campaigns against ACEs (1, 5). Reducing resource disparities in communities and providing additional services, including childcare and referrals to other programs, may also help reduce ACEs on a population level (6). However, research has shown that these types of primary prevention services are still relatively uncommon (6).

Secondary prevention measures can also be implemented, including early recognition and treatment of ACEs by pediatricians and other parties in a position to recognize and address them before further harm is incurred by the child (1). Increasing numbers of evidence-based secondary prevention measures are beginning to show promise, including parent-child interaction therapy and other types of interfamilial approaches (6). Screening for traumatic experiences can also be a useful tool to catch ACEs that were previously undiagnosed, but it has been shown to be underutilized among adolescents in health care settings (7).

TREATING ADVERSE CHILDHOOD EXPERIENCES

It is preferable to prevent ACEs before they occur, but this is not always possible. Fortunately, significant progress has been made in pursuit of treatment of ACEs. Cognitive behavior therapy (CBT) is among the leading treatment methods, and can be used for the whole family, which has been shown to be beneficial (6). A primary goal of CBT is to understand how trauma has affected them, and manage the feelings, thoughts, and behaviors stemming from that trauma (8).

As mentioned previously, screening for ACEs is increasingly being implemented in pediatric clinics and elsewhere, and can lead to early detection and treatment of ACEs (9). Although the type of treatment varies depending on the patient and the severity of their trauma, it has been speculated that the screening process itself can be therapeutic, functioning as an opportunity to talk about trauma and its potential effects on current health status (9).

EFFECTS OF ADVERSE CHILDHOOD EXPERIENCES ON ADOLESCENTS

It has already been documented that ACEs can increase depression and suicidal ideation, and this takes on an increased significance among adolescents, for whom suicide is one of the leading causes of mortality (10). Furthermore, strong associations have been shown between ACEs and susceptibility to mental health and substance use disorders, particularly among adolescents (11). All 10 categories of ACEs have been shown to increase early drug use initiation 2-4-fold, and increase likelihood of lifetime use (12). This can further complicate routine developmental and mental changes that occur during this period of life, and underscore the need for mental health and support services that are often lacking (7).

Adolescents who experienced trauma as children are also at increased risk of perpetrating violence, and the likelihood of this increases with ACE score (5). Compared to those with no ACEs, adolescent females with four or more ACEs show a 2-fold increase in bullying and 7-fold increase in suicide attempts, while males in the same category show a 4-fold increase in bullying and 10-fold increase in suicide attempts (5). Each type of adverse experience examined in this study, conducted Duke et al. (5) in 2010, showed significantly increased risk for violence-related outcomes; although results differed between male and female participants, results were significant for both groups5.

Recent research shows a dose-response relationship between ACE score and experience of violence in college, further implicating the life long impact of childhood trauma (13). A 2020 study by Cprek et al. found that among college students, those with an ACE score of 4 or more were between 1.9-4.9 times more likely to experience intimate partner violence (IPV) during college (13). Of the four types of violence examined (physical violence, psychological violence, sexual violence, and stalking), stalking was the most commonly reported, and was 4.9 times more common in the past 12 months among those with four or more ACEs (13).

TREATING TRAUMA

Until recent years, medical research has emphasized treatment of physical trauma (14). As diagnoses of post-traumatic stress disorder (PTSD) and other types of trauma have become more common, research on treatment methods for emotional and psychological trauma has increased (14).

Treating trauma is complex, and there is no one-size-fits-all solution. Researchers studying PTSD have proposed a framework for treatment comprised of three stages: 1) promoting safety, 2) processing traumatic memories and situational meanings and 3) restoring relationships and global meaning (4, 15). This process can give clinicians the freedom to work at the pace of the patient, and has shown promise in treating veterans suffering from PTSD (4).

Cognitive behavioral therapy (CBT) can be a useful tool, as discussed above. However, stored trauma can take root physiologically as well as psychologically, which has led to the development of the field of biology informed therapy (8). Biology informed therapy (BIT) seeks to help patients process traumatic experiences and reduce physiological response to stimuli, which may occur even when the patient has undergone CBT to process the psychological roots of trauma8. BIT can promote healing through connecting physical and emotional feeling and allowing healing on multiple levels (8).

TRAUMA-INFORMED CARE AND SUBSTANCE ABUSE

According to the Substance Abuse and Mental Health Services Administration (SAMHSA), trauma-informed care (also known as the trauma-informed approach) can be defined by the following:

> A program, organization, or system that is trauma-informed realizes the widespread impact of trauma and understands potential paths for recovery; recognizes the signs and symptoms of trauma in clients, families, staff, and others involved with the system; and responds by fully integrating knowledge about trauma into policies, procedures, and practices, and seeks to actively resist re-traumatization (16)

Trauma-informed care seeks to treat those with trauma, including those who are not aware that they have experienced trauma, without actively re-traumatizing them during the process (6). SAMHSA encourages those working in trauma-informed organizations to focus on the "Four R's": having basic realization of trauma and understanding how it can affect families, groups and communities in addition to individuals; recognizing signs of trauma as they appear by age, gender, and setting; responding by applying trauma-informed care principles in all areas of functioning; and resisting re-traumatization by understanding how patients have been affected by trauma (16). Additionally, SAMHSA promotes six key principles for a trauma-informed approach:

- Safety
- Trustworthiness and transparency
- Peer support
- Collaboration and mutuality

- Empowerment, voice, and choice
- Cultural, historical, and gender issues

By addressing these principles at multiple levels of organization, trauma can be addressed in a way that promotes efficient and productive healing (16).

In the past decade, there has been an increase in research linking trauma, physical health, behavioral health, and substance abuse (17). It has been documented that those who experienced trauma, as children or as adults, are predisposed to substance use disorders (SUDs) (17, 18). Child sexual abuse has also been linked with risky sexual acts and substance use, and potential sequelae include higher rates of infection with HIV and other STIs (18). Patients with a history of trauma often have worse SUD treatment outcomes (17), in part because their process of recovery is more difficult and nuanced, and the role of the counselor is more challenging (17). Thus, trauma-informed care can be a critical tool in treating these individuals (17).

Trauma-informed programs can use frameworks including the Social-Ecological Model to examine trauma across multiple levels, focusing on both risk factors and protective factors to isolate the effects of trauma and promote healing (16). Addressing this underlying trauma can facilitate recovery from SUDs (17) and hopefully break the cycle of trauma.

Conclusion

Adverse childhood experiences (ACEs) are common, highly interrelated, and commonly go undiagnosed. Untreated ACEs can lead to significant health effects later in life – among the most significant of these impacts is a 4- to 12-fold increase in risk for depression, suicide, and substance abuse (1). Data has shown that trauma increases risk for addiction and substance use disorder (SUD), sometimes as a means of comfort or self-treatment (2). Considering a trauma-informed care approach for those with SUD and other addiction disorders, particularly those with a history of ACEs, could change the treatment landscape and promote effective and long-lasting recovery.

REFERENCES

[1] Felitti VJ, Anda RF, Nordenberg D. Relationship of childhood abuse and household dysfunction to many of the leading causes of death in adults: The Adverse Childhood Experiences (ACE) Study. Am J Prev Med 2019;56(6):774-86.

[2] Covington SS. Women and addiction: A trauma-informed approach. J Psychoactive Drugs 2008;40(sup5):377-85.

[3] CDC. Prevention. Preventing adverse childhood experiences: Leveraging the best available evidence. Atlanta, GA: National Center for Injury Prevention and Control, Centers for Disease Control and Prevention, 2019.

[4] Carroll TD, Currier JM, McCormick WH, Drescher KD. Adverse childhood experiences and risk for suicidal behavior in male Iraq and Afghanistan veterans seeking PTSD treatment. Psychol Trauma 2017;9(5):583-6.

[5] Duke NN, Pettingell SL, McMorris BJ, Borowsky IW. Adolescent violence perpetration: associations with multiple types of adverse childhood experiences. Pediatrics 2010;125(4):e778-86.

[6] Oral R, Ramirez M, Coohey C. Adverse childhood experiences and trauma informed care: the future of health care. Pediatr Res 2016;79(1):227-33.

[7] Soleimanpour S, Geierstanger S, Brindis CD. Adverse childhood experiences and resilience: addressing the unique needs of adolescents. Acad Pediatrics 2017;17(7):S108-14.

[8] Solomon EP, Heide KM. The biology of trauma: Implications for treatment. J Interpers Violence 2005;20(1):51-60.

[9] Finkelhor D. Screening for adverse childhood experiences (ACEs): Cautions and suggestions. Child Abuse Neglect 2018;85:174-9.

[10] Curtin SC, Heron M, Miniño AM, Warner M. Recent increases in injury mortality among children and adolescents aged 10-19 years in the United States: 1999-2016. Natl Vital Stat Rep 2018;67(4):1-16.

[11] Somaini L, Donnini C, Manfredini M. Adverse childhood experiences (ACEs), genetic polymorphisms and neurochemical correlates in experimentation with psychotropic drugs among adolescents. Neurosci Biobehav Rev 2011;35(8):1771-8.

[12] Dube SR, Felitti VJ, Dong M, Chapman DP, Giles WH, Anda RF. Childhood abuse, neglect, and household dysfunction and the risk of illicit drug use: the adverse childhood experiences study. Pediatrics 2003;111(3):564-72.

[13] Cprek SE, Fisher BS, McDonald MJ, McDaniel HM, Williamson L, Williams CM. Adverse childhood experiences and interpersonal violence among college students:

does a relationship exist? J Am Coll Health 2020 Jan 29:1-8. doi: 10.1080/07448481.2020.1715413.
[14] Whitfield CL. Adverse childhood experiences and trauma. Am J Prev Med 1998;14(4):361-4.
[15] Herman JL. Trauma and recovery: The aftermath of violence from domestic abuse to political terror. New York: Basic Books, 1997.
[16] Substance Abuse and Mental Health Services Administration. Concept of trauma and guidance for a trauma-informed approach. Rockville, MD: SAMHSA, 2014.
[17] Substance Abuse and Mental Health Services Administration.Trauma-informed care in behavioral health services. Rockville, MD: SAMHSA, 2014.
[18] Ompad DC, Ikeda RM, Shah N. Childhood sexual abuse and age at initiation of injection drug use. Am J Public Health 2005;95(4):703-9.

In: Building Children and Youth for the Future ISBN: 978-1-53618-806-6
Editors: Joav Merrick et al.

Chapter 7

NEUROBIOLOGY OF SUICIDE

Kimberly Baran, DO, Brinda Ryali, Maria Demma Cabral*, MD and Dilip R Patel, MD, MBA, MPH
Department of Pediatric and Adolescent Medicine,
Western Michigan University Homer Stryker MD School of Medicine,
Kalamazoo, Michigan, United States of America

Suicide is a leading cause of death globally, especially in the adolescent population. A complex interplay of predisposing genetic and environmental factors in relation to abnormal biological processes contributes to the causation of suicide. There has been significant research conducted to discover the neurobiological processes that contribute to suicide. This chapter serves to review the key predisposing factors for suicide as well as provide insight into the developments of the neurobiological causes of suicide that have been uncovered.

* Corresponding Author's Email: mariademma.cabral@med.wmich.edu.

INTRODUCTION

Suicide claims the lives of approximately one million people annually and is an important phenomenon that has devastating cultural and socioeconomic implications (1). Significant research into the neurobiology of suicide and suicidal behavior has revealed many insights as to what makes an individual decide to go against their basic survival instincts and end their own lives. Many factors can predispose an individual to suicide such as genetics, early life adversity, and the acquired capability for suicide (ACS). Biologic abnormalities in the serotonergic system, hypothalamic-pituitary-adrenal (HPA) axis, and neuroimmune system have all been shown to play roles in the neurobiology of suicide as well as atypical activation of specific brain regions. Throughout this chapter, the term suicide will refer to all completed acts of purposely ending one's own life. Such acts that do not result in ending one's life, but were intended to do so, will be referred to as suicide attempts. Suicide behavior will describe all acts such as suicide, attempted suicide, and suicidal ideation and planning.

PUBLIC HEALTH PERSPECTIVE OF SUICIDE

Suicide is the 10th leading cause of death for all ages in the United States (1). Teenagers are at exponentially higher risk for suicide and suicidal behavior as compared to the general population, as suicide is the second leading cause of death in teenagers (1, 2). This may be because there are some psychosocial factors that are more common in this time of life, such as underdeveloped coping mechanisms, bullying, and peer victimization, that can contribute to suicidal behaviors. In 2017, 17% of high school students reported having had serious thoughts of attempting suicide, with females twice likely than males to do so having also reported more suicide attempts and needing medical attention for having attempted (3).

REVIEW OF PREDISPOSING AND RISK FACTORS FOR SUICIDE BEHAVIOR

Suicidal behavior has been found to be increased in individuals with mood and psychiatric disorders. Many of these disorders have genetic predisposition themselves, however, genetic predisposition to suicidal behavior may be somewhat independent from the genetic risk for psychiatric disorders (2). This claim was supported by an abundance of research involving families, twins, and adopted individuals. It is estimated that there is a heritability of suicide risk between 21-50% and of suicidal behavior between 30-55% (4). Vorecek et al. (4) claimed that there is a significantly higher concordance for suicidal behavior in monozygotic twins (24.1%), as compared to dizygotic twins (2.8%).

Trauma and early life adversity (ELA) are also believed to predispose individuals to suicidal behavior. Carballo et al. (5) noted that ELA includes events such as sexual or physical abuse, neglect, parental loss, or severe family discord. Both sexual and physical abuse have been shown to independently contribute to repeated suicide attempts, even after controlling for various other ELAs. Animal and human studies have shown lasting changes in the HPA axis and serotonergic and dopaminergic systems associated with ELA. It is thought that the long-term consequences of these changes include increased risk of developing a psychiatric disorder and behavioral traits such as aggression and impulsivity – all of which increases risk for suicidal behavior (5).

There are a few clinical traits that are repeatedly associated with suicidal behavior. As mentioned above, impulsivity is one of these traits. Impulsivity has been considered a familial trait according to Pandey et al. (2). This trait can put individuals at risk for suicide as it can cause them to act on their suicidal thoughts. Other traits include aggression, pessimism, and hopelessness. In fact, individuals with a history of attempting suicide had greater lifetime impulsivity and aggression than non-attempters when controlling for psychiatric illnesses (2).

Biologic Changes in Suicide

In the model proposed by Carballo, genetic predispositions and childhood adversities impact how the HPA axis responds to stress and interacts with neurohormones like norepinephrine, dopamine, and serotonin. These neurochemical and neuroendocrine makers in turn impact clinical endophenotypes such as impulsivity, aggression, pessimism, neuroticism, and hopelessness. An interplay of all three of these endophenotypes – clinical, neurochemical, and neuroendocrine, may play a causal role in the propensity to manifest suicidal behaviors or in impacting the probability of suicidal behavior (5).

The same authors identified the following associations between clinical endophenotypes and neurohormones. Increased impulsivity was associated with low 5-hydroxyindoleacetic acid in cerebrospinal fluid levels. Increased aggression was associated with low serotonergic activity, high norepinephrine concentrations, and increased dopamine concentrations. Of note, increased dopamine may be related to lethal suicidal behavior. Higher neuroticism scores were associated to the short variant of serotonin transporter linked polymorphic region and high density of striatal dopamine D2 receptors. Hopelessness was associated with changes in the serotonergic, where increased 5-Hydroxytryptamine 2A receptor activity resulted in decreased hopelessness. Rat studies have also shown that acquired helplessness is associated with changes in the norepinephrine system (5).

A similar review by Heeringen specified the three neurobiological systems and classified them as state-dependent (noradrenergic system and HPA axis) and trait-dependent (serotonergic system). Such characteristics has been suggested helpful in assessing risk and identifying prevention measures in suicidal behavior (6).

GENES AND SUICIDAL BEHAVIOR

Carballo et al. (5) examined multiple studies to report findings on genes that may be involved in suicidal behavior. Polymorphisms in serotonin transporter gene have been shown to result in fewer bindings sites, decreases serotonin function, and decreased neuro-hormonal response to citalopram in healthy individuals. Monoamine oxidase A (MAOA) gene polymorphisms have been associated with impulsivity and aggression. Polymorphisms that result in reduced MAOA expression have been associated with a history of early abuse in males. Given its location on the X chromosome, polymorphisms on this gene may contribute to the gender paradox of suicide behavior.

Tryptophan hydroxylase gene was shown to have increased mRNA expression in the dorsal and median raphe nuclei of the brainstem in suicides, most likely a compensatory response to decreased serotonin levels in suicide victims. Catechol-O-methyltransferase (COMT) polymorphisms have been reported to have a wide range of findings – from associations with violent suicide attempts seen in the Met allele to a protective role against suicide seen in the high activity Val/Val genotype (5).

ACQUIRED CAPABILITY FOR SUICIDE (ACS)

Desphande et al. attempted to explain the gender paradox of suicide by examining suicidal desire and ACS as two separate concepts with independent neural networks (7). The authors described ACS as a construct that explains why suicide victims are able to complete this task as opposed to their counterparts who attempted suicide. They explain that suicidal ideation and desire alone are not enough to allow one to be able to commit suicide. Through the use of activation likelihood estimate meta-analysis, they identified neural networks associated with ACS and suicidal desire.

Identification of intersecting areas of activation allowed for a proposed ACS-depression network that highlights the differences between male and female suicidal behaviors. The individual also must have fearlessness about death and a physical pain tolerance – together deemed the ACS – in order to complete suicide. It is thought that exposure to painful and provocative life experiences, such as combat exposure or impulsive/aggressive behaviors, results in desensitization to fear of death and/or physical pain, which in turn allows the capability for lethal self-harm (7).

The authors demonstrated that the ACS-depression network was more widespread in males, which may explain why men with suicidal desire may be more likely to have fatal outcomes than women with suicidal desire, as it is thought that men may have more exposure to these types of experiences, and thus higher ACS than women. Of note, the primary motor cortex and the dorsolateral prefrontal cortex were only activated in males. On the other hand, the female network activated more limbic structures. Exclusive activation of motor areas in males and emotional, limbic areas in females is hypothesized to contribute to the increased lethality of suicidal behavior in males compared to the increased prevalence of suicidal desire in females. The ACS-depression network seeds were then further examined by identifying axonal trajectories originating from this network. While the putamen was activated in male and female ACS-depression network seeds, axonal trajectories were very different. While projections from the male putamen fed into areas of motor and executive control, female projections were localized (7).

OTHER INTERESTING STUDIES

There had been studies correlating subjective sleep disturbances to suicidal ideation and behavior and use of sleep electroencephalography (EEG) has been a useful tool in biomarker identification. Dolsen et al. presented one of the first studies to look at quantitative sleep EEG as a neurobiological relation to suicidal ideation using a study population of adults with major depressive disorder (MDD). Results showed adults with MDD who reported higher suicidal ideation had hyperarousal during sleep demonstrated as increased electrophysiological brain activity (8).

More neuroimaging studies have been of interest in the study of suicide. One study presented an assessment of suicidal individuals using functional magnetic resonance imaging (fMRI) that helps identify altered neural signatures of concepts (8). Neurosematic analyses were performed on two groups: 17 suicidal ideators versus 17 healthy controls. The stimuli included 30 concepts each presented for three seconds and were related to either suicide, positive affect, or negative affect, then the brain locations were identified using the fMRI. Six of the concepts (death, cruelty, trouble, carefree, good, and praise) and five of the brain locations (left inferior parietal, left inferior frontal gyrus, left superior medial frontal, anterior cingulate, and right middle temporal regions) provided the most accurate discrimination between the two groups which clinically correlated showing meaningful differences between the individuals in the suicidal and control groups (9).

Conclusion

There have been many biologic studies that have allowed significant insight into the different neurobiological causes of suicide. These breakthroughs are important as they could lead to better methods of screening for high risk individuals as well as preventing those who are high risk from attempting or completing suicide. Early identification of those at risk for suicide could play a huge role in decreasing the rates of suicide as studies have shown that up to 83% of individuals who die by suicide have been in contact with a primary care physician within the year prior to their death. Suicide is a very complex, multi-dimensional phenomenon with many different biologic processes, as well as genetic and environmental factors, contributing to its cause. Understanding the neurobiological processes that contribute to suicide, such as alterations of the serotonergic system, HPA axis, and neuroimmune function, could not only lead to methods of improved screening and early detection, but potentially targeted therapies.

REFERENCES

[1] Suicide. National Institute of Mental Health, 2019. URL: https://www.nimh.nih.gov/health/statistics/suicide.shtml.

[2] Pandey GN. Biological basis of suicide and suicidal behavior. Bipolar Disord 2013;15(5):524-41.

[3] Teen suicide. Child Trends Databank, 2019. URL: https://www.childtrends.org/?indicators=suicidal-teens.

[4] Padurariu M, Prepelita R, Ciobica A, Dobrin R, Timofte D, Stefanescu C, et al. Concept of suicide: neurophysiological/genetic theories and possible oxytocin relevance. Neurophys 2016;48(4):312-9.

[5] Carballo JJ, Currier D, Figueroa AE, Giner L, Kelly SA, Sublette ME, et al. Neurobiological underpinnings of suicidal behavior: Integrating data from clinical and biological studies. Eur J Psychiat 2009;23(4):243-59.

[6] Heeringen KV. The neurobiology of suicide and suicidality. Can J Psychiatry 2003;48(5):292-300.

[7] Deshpande G, Baxi M, Witte T, Robinson JL. A neural basis for the acquired capability for suicide. Front Psychiatry 2016;7:1-17.

[8] Dolsen MR, Cheng P, Arnedt JT, Swanson K, Casement MD, Kim HS, et al. Neurophysiological correlates of suicidal ideation in major depressive disorder: Hyperarousl during sleep. J Affect Disord 2017;212:160-6.

[9] Just MA, Pan L, Cherkassky VL, McMakin DL, Cha C, Nock MK, et al. Machine learning of neural representations of suicide and emotion concepts identifies suicidal youth. Nature Hum Behehav 2017;1:911-9.

In: Building Children and Youth for the Future ISBN: 978-1-53618-806-6
Editors: Joav Merrick et al.

Chapter 8

THE OLAMIND SCREENING TOOL FOR AUTISM SPECTRUM DISORDER IN CHILDREN AGED 4–18 YEARS

Rachelle Lavi**, *MSc
Independent Practice, Mazkeret Batya, Israel

ABSTRACT

Autism spectrum disorder (ASD) is a common neurodevelopmental condition whose diagnosis is often delayed. The feasibility of OlaMind, a new digital system to screen for ASD in verbal children and adolescents without intellectual disability, was tested. Parents in Israel used the instrument concerning their 4–18-year-old children with a doctor-given ASD diagnosis (ASD group: n = 33; 7 females) or without one (Control: n = 44; 20 females). A high proportion of the control group had parent-reported diagnoses of non-ASD conditions whose symptoms may resemble those of ASD (Other: n = 24; 9 females). Those who did not have such diagnoses were considered typically developing (TD: n = 20; 11 females). The algorithm classified 32 (97%) of ASD cases as

* *Correspondence:* Alex J Rachelle Singer Lavi (Rachelle Lavi), Independent Practice, PO Box 3186, Mazkeret Batya, 7680400, Israel. Email: lavirachelle@gmail.com.

exhibiting an ASD symptom pattern across DSM-5 clinical diagnostic domains and one 18-year-old male as exhibiting a non-ASD symptom pattern. The algorithm classified 75% of TD cases and 50% of Other cases as non-ASD. There was good correlation between the analytic groups and algorithm classifications. Two Other cases and one TD case were subsequently diagnosed with ASD or with multiple other conditions, respectively. Classification accuracy, sensitivity, and specificity were 78%, 97%, and 67%, respectively, in the full sample; 91%, 94%, and 89%, respectively, for the ASD and TD groups; and 93%, 94%, and 92%, respectively for the ASD and TD groups after accounting for subsequent known diagnoses. The results demonstrate the feasibility of the OlaMind algorithm. A full validation and reliability study is planned.

INTRODUCTION

Autism spectrum disorder (ASD) is a neurodevelopmental condition that is diagnosed clinically by the presence of pervasive deficits in social interaction and communication combined with restricted, repetitive interests (1, 2). The clinical ASD phenotype exhibits considerable heterogeneity, and ASD occurs without comorbid intellectual disability in about 40% of children and adolescents (3). Once considered a rare condition (4), childhood ASD prevalence estimates of around 1% are now common in diverse locations (5–7).

Considerable effort is made to diagnose children with ASD prior to age three years. Nevertheless, in the United States (US), a third to nearly a half of children (depending on ethnicity) receive their ASD diagnosis only after age five years (3). Indeed, even optimal screening of very young children is likely to miss some, because deficits in the use of language for social purposes (i.e., in pragmatic language) generally cannot be diagnosed prior to age 4–5 years (8). As some children are initially able to compensate for their pragmatic language difficulties, a presentation clearly consistent with ASD may only evolve at older ages (9).

In addition to child-related variables, late diagnosis may also reflect delays in health-provider response to parental concerns (10, 11). Even in developed countries, pediatricians and/or family doctors often require better training in child development (12). Complicating the physician's task, there are several conditions that share symptom overlap with ASD or whose symptoms are similar to those of ASD. Individuals with social (pragmatic) communication disorder (SCD) exhibit deficits in social communication. Although SCD does not also include restricted, repetitive behavior patterns, the nature of core symptom overlap between SCD and ASD is such that the diagnostic criteria laid out in the fifth edition of the "Diagnostic and statistical manual of mental disorders (DSM-5)" for SCD specifically direct the physician to consider whether the symptoms "are not better explained by autism spectrum disorder" (2).

Attention-deficit/hyperactivity disorder (ADHD) is a common developmental condition among school-aged children (13, 14). Although the core symptoms of ADHD (inattention, hyperactivity, and impulsivity) do not overlap with those of ASD, they frequently co-occur (15), and children with ADHD often have social and adaptation difficulties that resemble those seen in ASD, such that their diagnostic differentiation can be very challenging (16). There is also the potential for diagnostic confusion and considerable levels of comorbidity between ASD and anxiety (17), obsessive compulsive disorder (OCD) (18), Tourette's disorder (19), and other conditions (20).

Screening clinicians' confidence that a child may have ASD appears to guide their decision-making regarding whether to refer that child for full diagnostic assessment, with confidence in turn dependent on parent-reported unusual behaviors (21). Complex presentations and mild cases are particularly likely to experience clinician-related delays in obtaining ASD diagnosis (22). Consistently with this, children with additional diagnoses receive their ASD diagnosis significantly later than children without them (23) and children and adolescents with IQ $\geq$ 85 have a much longer pathway to ASD diagnosis than those with a lower IQ (10).

The difficulty in diagnosing ASD affects families. A retrospective examination of Israeli cases found that 221 children diagnosed with ASD after age 6 years underwent 1,028 developmental evaluations prior to age 6 years (9). Parents in Germany have been found to consult up to 20 different professionals until their child receives an ASD diagnosis (10). Parents in the US describe the diagnostic process for ASD as "arduous, lengthy, and fraught with difficulties" (24).

When a long period elapses from when developmental concerns are first raised until the achievement of correct diagnosis, the provision of appropriate treatment is delayed. Earlier intervention raises the likelihood of improved developmental trajectory (25, 26) and, indeed, delayed diagnosis is associated with worse outcomes for the affected individual (27) and increased costs to the family (28) and, presumably, to publicly-funded health systems.

Rationale

As described above, ASD is a common condition whose diagnosis is complex and often delayed for a variety of reasons to the detriment of affected individuals, their families, and the public health system. It is not realistic to expect all children with ASD to be diagnosed as such in early childhood, thus research and clinical efforts need to focus also on later periods.

It is proposed that navigation of the pre-diagnostic period for individuals aged four years and over with undiagnosed ASD could be improved by addressing: 1) the quality of parental reports of their child's behavior to health practitioners in the community and 2) parent–clinician communication, in general, and referral-related decision-making, in particular. Parent-report rather than clinician insight is the first point of focus out of a belief that there is more scope for improvement in this area. Specifically, it may be easier to improve parents' descriptions of their children's behavior than to provide non-specialist community clinicians with training in child development sufficient to enable them to suspect ASD in verbal children without intellectual disability during a short consultation with parents whose concerns are often incomplete, disorganized and very unspecific. This provides the basis for the second point of focus, namely, to improve communication between parents and community health practitioners and support the clinician's referral-related decision-making in the current diagnostic environment, which is defined by the DSM-5 (2) and by the less prescriptive eleventh revision of the "International classification of diseases" (ICD-11) (1).

Existing screening instruments intended for use with older children in a community context are of limited utility for various reasons. The current Gilliam Rating Scales (GARS-3) has not yet been independently examined, however its earlier versions were found to have limited clinical utility (29). The Childhood Autism Spectrum Test (CAST; 30), which was developed about a decade prior to the DSM-5, does not appear to fully reflect the current diagnostic environment and, having been designed for use with 5–11 year olds, does not cover adolescence. The publisher of the Autism Spectrum Rating Scales (the ASRS) and the Social Responsiveness Scale (the SRS-II) limits the availability of both instruments via qualification restrictions that would exclude most parents (31).

The development of a new screening tool could contribute to increased community accessibility to DMS-5-consistent ASD screening and improved communication between parents and health practitioners, as the basis for more appropriate differential diagnostic assessment. To that end, I developed a system to screen for ASD comprehensively and in a balanced manner according to the clinical diagnostic criteria of the DSM-5 (2). The system comprises a digital ASD questionnaire, scoring algorithm, and report, with the latter designed to improve communication between parents and health practitioners and support clinical decision-making regarding referral to specialist assessment (where indicated). Upon conclusion of the study, the system was named OlaMind, and it is referred to as such throughout this paper.

The current study aimed to examine the feasibility of the OlaMind algorithm by conducting a preliminary assessment of its ability to classify children and adolescents with and without ASD prior to undertaking a larger, statistically robust study.

Methods

A case-control design was adopted, in which the detection of children and adolescents with a diagnosis of ASD (the ASD group) was compared with the detection of those without a diagnosis of ASD (Controls). Data were obtained from parent participants (the respondents) who served as proxies with respect to their 4–18-year-old children (the cases).

Participants

The parents or guardians of children and adolescents aged 4–18 years who were verbal and did not have an intellectual disability (ID) were eligible to participate. Participants were recruited over a 50-day period in early 2018 by a snowball technique driven by word of mouth and messaging on social media.

Instruments

Both instruments used in this research were initially constructed in English. They were then translated into Hebrew by a professional translator with a social sciences background. The translations were then checked for accuracy, clarity, and retention of similar language by a native Hebrew speaker fluent in English together with the researcher. Corrections were made as necessary, with disagreements resolved by consensus. The instruments were then programmed as components of an Android™ application.

Procedure

Participants were asked to download the app from GooglePlay™ to any Android device and use it with respect to their own children. The user could choose English or Hebrew as the display language. The first screen of the app provided a general description of the tool and its privacy provisions, whose active acceptance was required in order to continue, such that all participation was on an active opt-in basis.

The demographic questionnaire was then displayed followed by the index OlaMind questionnaire. Upon conclusion of the last OlaMind questionnaire item, participants pressed “send,” the algorithm analyzed the data, with the data were transmitted to a secure FireBase™ database. The next screen requested permission to contact the participant for follow-up, again on an opt-in basis. The final screen presented the results report.

Demographic questionnaire

The demographic questionnaire asked for the child or adolescent’s name and sex (male/female). The questionnaire referred to the child by name to help focus the respondent. Hebrew does not possess gender-neutral nouns, pronouns, verbs, or modifiers, with communication in the Hebrew language requiring the use of either ‘male’ or ‘female’ language. The child’s sex was used not only to characterize the sample, but also to determine whether the child would be referred to in male or female Hebrew in the OlaMind questionnaire.

Participants were then asked for the child’s date of birth. The digital instrument prevented data entry concerning cases whose dates of birth indicated age of less than 4 years or of 19 or more years. Birth date was also used by the OlaMind questionnaire to determine which examples to display. Additional questions asked whether or not the child speaks in sentences, and the respondent’s relationship to the child.

For the purpose of grouping the cases for analysis, respondents were also asked: Has a doctor told you that the child has any of the following: Anxiety/ depression/emotional problems; attention deficit (hyperactivity) disorder (ADHD); autism spectrum disorder (ASD, autism, Asperger's, pervasive developmental disorder (PDD)); intellectual disability; learning disability; obsessive compulsive disorder (OCD); Tourette's or other tic disorder; schizophrenia or other psychosis; none of the above. These conditions were selected because they are frequently the initial diagnostic impression in children who are subsequently diagnosed with ASD, their symptoms resemble those of ASD, or they can be mistaken for it (9, 20, 32, 33). By oversight, SCD was omitted from the list of diagnoses. The app was programmed to enable respondents to advance from screen to screen only if all questions were answered.

OlaMind questionnaire

The questionnaire consisted of 30 items and was presented one item per screen. The items were presented in a pseudo-randomized order defined using a list randomizer (https://www.random.org/lists/). Respondents could only submit the questionnaire if a response was recorded for all items, with respondents directed to complete items with missing responses.

Each item consisted of a statement and examples, which exemplified how the statement could manifest in daily life. Eighteen items were written to represent DMS-5 ASD criteria A1–3 and another 12 were written to represent DSM-5 ASD criteria B1–4. This matches the 3:2 ratio of ASD criterion A to criterion B in the DSM-5 (2), and so reflects the greater weight given by the DSM-5 clinical diagnostic criteria to social communication symptoms.

The respondent was asked to agree or disagree with each statement. The ASD-typical response was variously agree or disagree, but was always encoded as 1 (nominal dichotomous). A mentioned above, date of birth determined the examples used to illustrate the OlaMind questionnaire's statements. There were three age ranges for the examples: 4–8 years; 9–12 years; and 13–18 years. These age ranges were chosen to take into account pubertal, neuro- and social-development.

The average age of pubertal onset is at 9–10 years in females and males (34). At around this age, more adult-like specialization of the brain regions involved in reasoning about others' minds (i.e., theory of mind; ToM) also occurs, with correct ToM behaviors measured in about 80–

100% of tested instances by age 8 years and improving through to age 12 years (35). Consequently, the youngest age group was defined as 4–8 years. Adolescence is marked by distinctly different social behaviors compared with juvenility (36). Consequently, the older two age groups were defined as 9–12 years (which corresponds to pubertal onset) and 13–18 years (which corresponds to adolescence).

A check box beside each example allowed respondents to indicate examples applying to their child. Furthermore, respondents could add their own comments or child-specific examples in free text beneath each item.

Feedback

All parents could choose to submit written feedback via a feedback field. Parents were asked if they authorized contact and those who did so were later e-mailed seeking permission to phone them to discuss their experience using the app, asked for a phone number for that purpose, and also given the researcher's phone number. Only those who chose to reply to the e-mail were then contacted by phone. Feedback data were utilized for data control but are not analyzed herein.

Data analysis

Data were downloaded from FireBase for analysis as a single consolidated JavaScript Object Notation (JSON) file, which was then converted to Excel® for analysis. The OlaMind algorithm classified each case on the basis of parent responses to the OlaMind items. Spearman's correlations were calculated to compare the analytical groups with the algorithm's assignations. Significance was set to .05. The classification accuracy, sensitivity, and specificity of the OlaMind instrument were also calculated. Figure 1 shows flow through the study, and the age ranges and male to female ratios in each group.

Algorithm classifications

The proprietary OlaMind algorithm was designed to classify a very wide range of response patterns consolidated into broad groups. Classification A was intended to capture cases showing a DSM-5-compatible ASD symptom pattern, with cases in this category exhibiting, frankly or in a borderline manner, communication symptoms from across DSM-5 section A. Classifications B and C were intended to capture non-ASD cases. Classification B was programmed to capture cases showing ASD symptoms whose pattern suggested that they do not arise from ASD, in that they do not show even a borderline DSM-5-consistent symptom pattern. Classification C was intended to capture cases showing few or no ASD symptoms (2).

Analytical groups

The analytical groups were formed on the basis of responses to questions as to whether the child or adolescent had any of the diagnoses referred to in the demographic questionnaire, with multiple responses or a "none of the above" response permitted. The ASD group comprised children and adolescents whose parent had ticked the presence of "Autism Spectrum Disorder (ASD, autism, Asperger's, or pervasive developmental disorder (PDD))" with or without comorbidities. The Control group comprised children and adolescents whose parent had ticked one or more of the six non-ASD non-intellectual disability diagnoses covered by the demographic questionnaire (intellectual disability being an exclusion criterion) or "none of the above." In this study, no parents endorsed their child having schizophrenia or another psychosis. One parent who ticked the ASD box and then added a comment that the child actually had SCD was also included in this group.

The algorithm classifications were then compared with the analytical groups. If the algorithm performed as expected, then it would: (1) assign

ASD group members to Classification A; and (2) assign Control group members to either of the non-ASD Classifications B or C.

RESULTS

Data were received from mothers concerning 74 cases and from fathers concerning six cases, for a total of 80 children and adolescents. Data concerning two adolescents with ID (an exclusion criterion) were excluded prior to data analysis. Careless responses may be removed from data to avoid contaminating their analysis (37). One adolescent was therefore excluded prior to data analysis after his mother stated (during a follow-up interview) that she had responded carelessly. Overall, data were analyzed concerning 77 children and adolescents aged 4.0–18.9 years

On the basis of answers to the question about diagnoses, the cases were grouped to the ASD (n = 33; 7 females; age range 5.0–17.5 years; mean age, 10.7 years; SD 3.9) and Control groups (n = 44; 20 females; age range 4.4–18.9 years; mean age, 11.2 years; SD 3.9). The age groups were evenly distributed in the ASD group (11 individuals in each of the 4–8, 9–12, and 13–18-year age groups) and reasonably distributed in the Control group (13, 17, and 14 individuals in the 4–8, 9–12, and 13–18-year age groups, respectively). Over half the Control group had a reported diagnosis of non-ASD 'other' condition(s). This proportion is much higher than that in the general child and adolescent population, for which the highest-prevalence conditions (among those considered here) are ADHD (estimated prevalence, 9.5%) and learning disabilities (estimated prevalence, 7.7%) (38). Therefore, the Control group was further subdivided into Other and typically developing (TD) groups. Children and adolescents with a respondent-reported diagnosis of any of the non-ASD conditions listed in the demographic questionnaire were placed in the Other group (n = 24; 9 females; age range 4.4–18.0 years; mean age, 12.2 years; SD 4.0). Those with no respondent-reported diagnoses were placed in the TD group (n = 20; 11 females; age range 4.0–18.9 years; mean age, 9.7 years; SD 3.6). The between-group difference in mean age was not significant for the ASD and Other groups (t = 1.418, df = 55, p = .16) but was significant for the TD and Other groups (t = 2.159, df = 42, p = .018).

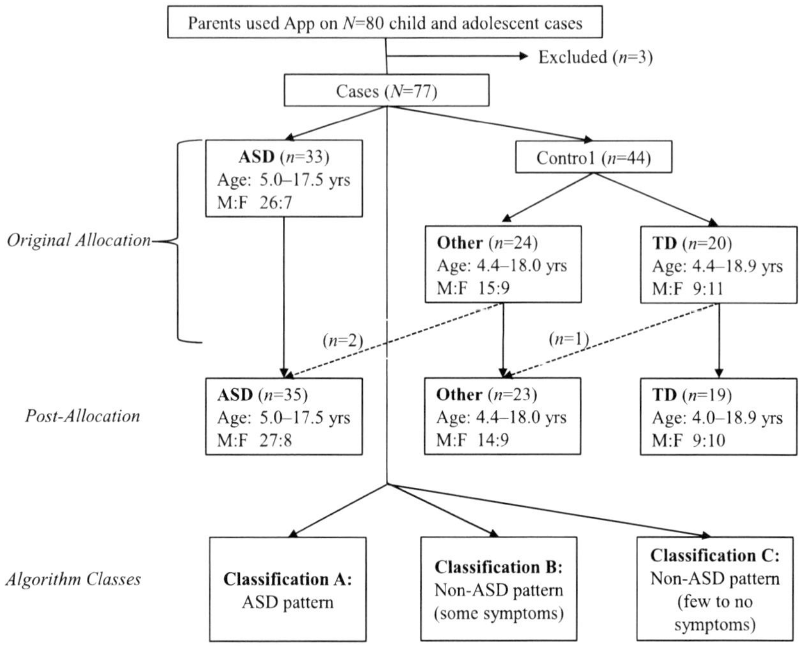

Figure 1. Flow through the study. As a result of diagnostic assessments conducted after respondents used OlaMind, some cases moved between groups, as shown by the dashed arrows.

One respondent subsequently contacted the researcher. She had used OlaMind while two of her children were waitlisted for ASD assessment. At the request of the ASD assessment center, a third sibling was also assessed. Following these assessments, two of the children (who were in the Other group at the time of data collection) were diagnosed with ASD and another (who was in the TD group at the time of data collection) received non-ASD diagnoses. Taking this information into account, the post-allocation groups (see Figure 1) were therefore: ASD (n = 35; 8 females; age range 5.0–17.5 years; mean age, 10.8 years; SD 3.9); Other (n = 23; 9 females; age range 4.4–18.0 years; mean age, 12.1 years; SD 3.9); and TD (n = 19; 10 females; age range 4.0–18.9 years; mean age, 9.6 years; SD 3.6). The post-allocation between-group difference in mean age was not significant for the ASD and Other groups ($t = 1.214$, $df = 56$, $p = .11$) or for the ASD and TD groups ($t = 1.109$, $df = 52$, $p = .14$) but was significant for the TD and Other groups ($t = 2.14$, $df=40$, $p = .019$).

Performance of the algorithm

The performance of the algorithm was examined with respect to the allocations made based on diagnoses reported at the time of data collection (see Figure 2A) and on the basis of the revised allocations made after taking into account diagnoses known to have been made subsequently (see Figure 2B).

Performance vis-à-vis original allocation

As shown in Figure 2A, of the 33 children and adolescents with a reported diagnosis of ASD at the time of data collection, the algorithm classified 32 (97%) to Classification A, as expected, and one 18-year-old male (3%) to non-ASD Classification B.

Nearly two thirds (n = 28; 64%) of the 44 children and adolescents who were in the Control group at the time of data collection were classified by the algorithm to one of the non-ASD classifications (Classifications B or C), as expected. About a third (n = 16, 32%) were assigned to Classification A. Three quarters (75%) of these Classification A assignations involved children or adolescents who had been diagnosed with a condition whose symptoms overlap with or may resemble those of ASD.

Of the 24 children and adolescents in the Other group, the algorithm assigned 12 (50%) to a non-ASD classification (5 to Classification B; 7 to Classification C), as expected, and the other 12 to Classification A (Figure 2A). The algorithm assigned 16 (75%) of the 20 TD group children and adolescents to Classification C, as expected, while assigning four (25%) to

Classification A (Figure 2A). Of these four, one subsequently received two diagnoses from the list of those queried by the demographic questionnaire. No information was available for the other three, whose parents endorsed numerous symptoms across all three DSM-5 ASD Section A domains and across 2–4 ASD Section B domains.

When the Control group as a whole was analyzed by number of other diagnoses, a trend emerged between the number of such diagnoses and algorithm classification. The greater the number of other diagnoses, the greater the percentage of cases assigned to Classification A by the algorithm (Figure 3A).

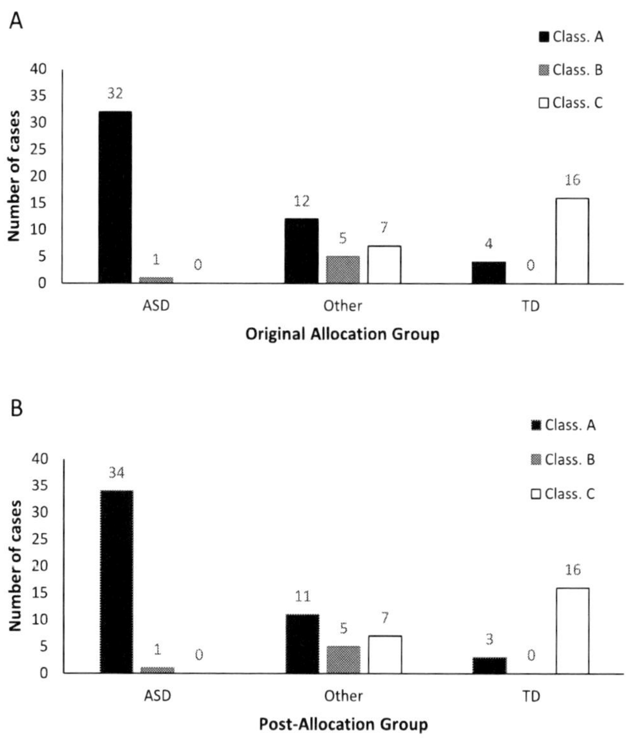

Figure 2. Performance of the algorithm. Algorithm assignment to ASD classification A and to non-ASD classifications B and C for the ASD, other, and typically developing (TD) groups. (A) On the basis of diagnoses reported at the time of data collection (original allocation groups). (B) Taking into account diagnoses made after using OlaMind (post-allocation groups).

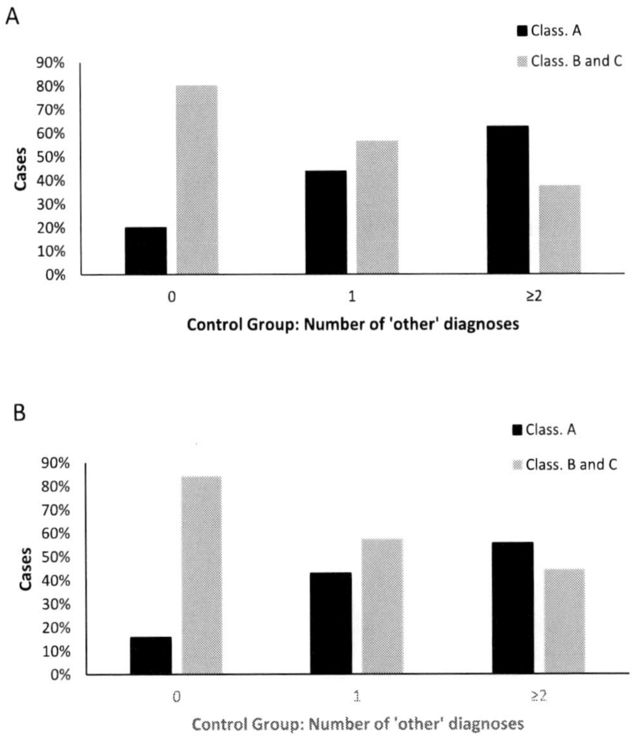

Figure 3. Relationship between the number of other diagnoses and algorithm-assigned classification within the control group. As the number of other diagnoses reported for a child or adolescent increased, so too did the percentage of cases that the algorithm assigned to ASD classification A compared with non-ASD classifications B or C. Control group cases had parent-reported other diagnoses of: anxiety, depression, or emotional problems; attention deficit (hyperactivity) disorder, learning disability; obsessive compulsive disorder; and/or Tourette's or other tic disorder.

For the total sample, the Spearman's correlation between the three analytic groups and the three algorithm classifications was good ($r(76) = .70$, $p = <.00001$). The Spearman's correlation improved when only the ASD and TD groups were considered ($r(52) = .84$, $p = <.00001$). Calculations for ASD versus Control yielded classification accuracy 77.9%, sensitivity 96.6%, and specificity 66.7%. These values improved when only the ASD and TD groups were considered: classification accuracy 90.6%, sensitivity 94.1%, and specificity 88.9%.

Performance vis-à-vis post-allocation

Post-allocation, the size of the ASD group increased from 33 to 35 individuals, whereas the control group decreased from 44 to 42 members (see Figure 1). As was seen in the original allocation data, the greater the number of other diagnoses, the greater the percentage of cases assigned to classification A (see Figure 3B). For the total sample, the Spearman's correlation was good ($r(76) = .74$, $p = <.00001$). The Spearman's correlation improved when only the ASD and TD groups were considered ($r(53) = .87$, $p= <.00001$). Calculations for ASD versus Control yielded classification accuracy 80.5%, sensitivity 96.6%, and specificity 70.8%. These values improved when only the ASD and TD groups were considered: classification accuracy 92.6%, sensitivity 94.1%, and specificity 91.9%.

Discussion

The OlaMind algorithm was developed to differentiate between children and adolescents with and without ASD, as defined by the clinical diagnostic criteria of the DSM-5 (2). Methods to detect developmental problems are typically assessed in terms of their sensitivity, being the proportion of individuals with a condition who are correctly identified as having it, and their specificity, being the proportion of individuals without a condition who are correctly identified as not having it. For screening tools intended for use in a primary care setting and relying on information from parents, suggested sensitivity and specificity standards are 70–80%, where specificity should preferably be closer to 80% to minimize over-referral (39).

In the preliminary study reported here and involving a small sample of 77 children and adolescents aged 4–18 years, the OlaMind algorithm accurately classified 78% of participants, with high sensitivity (97%) but with specificity (67%) lower than the target of around 80% (39). The diagnostically most challenging group of children and adolescents comprises those who present with symptoms found not only in ASD but also in other conditions. Under such circumstances, the aim of the referring physician is generally to suggest the most likely directions for the diagnosing specialist to consider as part of a differential diagnostic assessment. Children and adolescents presenting with such symptoms may already have one or more developmental or mental health diagnoses, which the diagnosing clinician may confirm, reject (in the event of earlier misdiagnosis), or add to (in the event of earlier partial diagnosis). The latter two circumstances need not imply previous clinician error, as presentation may change to become clearly ASD-suggestive only as children develop (9). Thus, the diagnostic picture for this clinical population is often far from clear. Consistently with this, it was found that 21% and 30% of children who were ultimately diagnosed with ADHD met ASD cutoffs on the Autism Diagnostic Observation Schedule (ADOS) and the Autism Diagnostic Interview-Revised (ADI-R), respectively (40). Similarly, 36% of clinically anxious children were found to meet at least one ADI-R cutoff and 31% were found to lie in the ASD range for current ASD behaviors (17). Therefore, the low specificity of OlaMind with respect to the total sample may reflect the high proportion of Control children with non-ASD diagnoses. The proportion of Control children and adolescents classified by the algorithm as ASD (i.e., Classification A) increased with increasing numbers of other reported diagnoses, which further supports this understanding.

When solely the ASD and TD groups were considered, classification accuracy rose to 91%, sensitivity dropped slightly to 94%, and specificity rose to 89%. After accounting for known diagnoses made after using OlaMind, classification accuracy further improved to 93%, sensitivity remained unchanged, and specificity rose to an excellent 92%. Although these figures may be overly high for use in a primary care setting (39), they indicate the strong potential of the OlaMind screening method and they support further development of the tool and continuation to an appropriately powered study of OlaMind's validity and reliability.

Conclusion

Initial testing of the OlaMind screening system on parent-provided data concerning 77 children and adolescents revealed good correlation between parent-reported ASD or non-ASD diagnosis and the algorithm's classifications of cases as ASD or non-ASD. The study had two main limitations. First, it was too small to permit generalization, and thus the results should be regarded as indicative. Second, the absence of follow-up of those who screened positive meant that, although one initially TD child was later diagnosed with other conditions and two children with other conditions were later diagnosed with ASD, it was not possible to investigate whether this occurred in other cases. Nevertheless, the results indicate that OlaMind exhibits high accuracy, sensitivity, and specificity, so supporting continuation to a full validity and reliability study with a larger sample.

Acknowledgment

The researcher thanks Professor Mark A. Stokes (Deakin University) for his insightful comments and guidance, professor Ditzah Zachor (Shamir Medical Center) and professor Esther Ben-Itzchak (Ariel University) for advice during the very early development of the instrument, and professor Cory Shulman (Hebrew University of Jerusalem) for her encouragement.

References

[1] World Health Organization. Mental, behavioural or neurodevelopmental disorders. In: International classification of diseases for mortality and morbidity statistics, 11th ed. Geneva: World Health Organization, 2018.

[2] American Psychiatric Association. Diagnostic and statistical manual of mental disorders, 5th ed. Washington, DC: American Psychiatric Association, 2013.

[3] Jo H, Schieve LA, Rice CE, Yeargin-Allsopp M, Tian LH, Blumberg SJ, et al. Age at autism spectrum disorder (ASD) diagnosis by race, ethnicity, and primary

household language among children with special health care needs, United States, 2009–2010. Matern Child Health J 2015;19(8):1687–97.

[4] Blaxill MF. What's going on? The question of time trends in autism. Public Health Rep 2004;119(6):536–51.

[5] Alshaban F, Aldosari M, Al-Shammari H, El-Hag S, Ghazal I, Tolefat M, et al. Prevalence and correlates of autism spectrum disorder in Qatar: a national study. J Child Psychol Psychiatry 2019;60(12):1254–68.

[6] Morales-Hidalgo P, Roigé-Castellví J, Hernández-Martínez C, Voltas N, Canals J. Prevalence and characteristics of autism spectrum disorder among Spanish school-age children. J Autism Dev Disord 2018;48(9):3176–90.

[7] Sun X, Allison C, Wei L, Matthews FE, Auyeung B, Wu YY, et al. Autism prevalence in China is comparable to Western prevalence. Mol Autism 2019;10(1):7.

[8] Swineford LB, Thurm A, Baird G, Wetherby AM, Swedo S. Social (pragmatic) communication disorder: a research review of this new DSM-5 diagnostic category. J Neurodev Disord 2014;6(1):41.

[9] Davidovitch M, Levit-Binnun N, Golan D, Manning-Courtney P. Late diagnosis of Autism Spectrum Disorder after initial negative assessment by a multidisciplinary team. J Dev Behav Pediatr 2015 May;36(4):227–34.

[10] Höfer J, Hoffmann F, Kamp-Becker I, Poustka L, Roessner V, Stroth S, et al. Pathways to a diagnosis of autism spectrum disorder in Germany: a survey of parents. Child Adolesc Psychiatry Ment Health 2019;13(1):16.

[11] Ozonoff S, Young GS, Brian J, Charman T, Shephard E, Solish A, et al. Diagnosis of autism spectrum disorder after age 5 in children evaluated longitudinally since infancy. J Am Acad Child Adolesc Psychiatry 2018;57(11):849-57.

[12] Tassone MC, Jegathesan T, Han R, Atkinson A, Ng S, Young E. Gaps in developmental pediatrics training: a Canadian resident physician perspective. MedEdPublish 2018;7(2):68–81.

[13] Polanczyk G V., Salum GA, Sugaya LS, Caye A, Rohde LA. Annual Research review: a meta-analysis of the worldwide prevalence of mental disorders in children and adolescents. J Child Psychol Psychiatry 2015;56(3):345–65.

[14] Thomas R, Sanders S, Doust J, Beller E, Glasziou P. Prevalence of attention-deficit/hyperactivity disorder: A systematic review and meta-analysis. Pediatrics 2015;135(4):e994–1001.

[15] Ronald A, Larsson H, Anckarsäter H, Lichtenstein P. Symptoms of autism and ADHD: A Swedish twin study examining their overlap. J Abnorm Psychol 2014;123(2):440–51.

[16] Salley B, Gabrielli J, Smith CM, Braun M. Do communication and social interaction skills differ across youth diagnosed with autism spectrum disorder, attention-deficit/hyperactivity disorder, or dual diagnosis? Res Autism Spectr Disord 2015;20:58–66.

[17] Van Steensel FJA, Bögels SM, Wood JJ. Autism spectrum traits in children with anxiety disorders. J Autism Dev Disord 2013;43:361–70.

[18] Griffiths DL, Farrell LJ, Waters AM, White SW. ASD traits among youth with Obsessive–Compulsive Disorder. Child Psychiatry Hum Dev 2017;48(6):911–21.

[19] Darrow SM, Grados M, Sandor P, Hirschtritt ME, Illmann C, Osiecki L, et al. Autism spectrum symptoms in a Tourette's disorder sample. J Am Acad Child Adolesc Psychiatry 2017;56(7):610-617.e1.

[20] Simms MD. When autistic behavior suggests a disease other than classic autism. Pediatr Clin North Am 2017;64(1):127–38.

[21] Hedley D, Brewer N, Nevill R, Uljarevic M, Butter E, Mulick JA. The relationship between clinicians' confidence and accuracy, and the influence of child characteristics, in the screening of autism spectrum disorder. J Autism Dev Disord 2016;46(7):2340–8.

[22] Gibbs V, Aldridge F, Sburlati E, Chandler F, Smith K, Cheng L. Missed opportunities: An investigation of pathways to autism diagnosis in Australia. Res Autism Spectr Disord 2019;57:55–62.

[23] Brett D, Warnell F, McConachie H, Parr JR. Factors affecting age at ASD diagnosis in UK: no evidence that diagnosis age has decreased between 2004 and 2014. J Autism Dev Disord 2016;46(6):1974–84.

[24] Oswald DP, Haworth SM, Mackenzie BK, Willis JH. Parental report of the diagnostic process and outcome: ASD compared with other developmental disabilities. Focus Autism Other Dev Disabl 2017;32(2):152–60.

[25] Koegel LK, Koegel RL, Ashbaugh K, Bradshaw J. The importance of early identification and intervention for children with or at risk for autism spectrum disorders. Int J Speech Lang Pathol 2014;16(1):50–6.

[26] Wood S, Christian MP, Sampson A. Audit of outcomes following a community-based early intensive behaviour intervention program for children with autism in Australia. Aust J Psychol 2018;70(3):217–24.

[27] Heeramun R, Magnusson C, Gumpert CH, Granath S, Lundberg M, Dalman C, et al. Autism and convictions for violent crimes: population-based cohort study in Sweden. J Am Acad Child Adolesc Psychiatry 2017;56(6):491-7.

[28] Horlin C, Falkmer M, Parsons R, Albrecht MA, Falkmer T. The cost of autism spectrum disorders. PLoS One 2014;9(9):e106552.

[29] Pandolfi V, Magyar CI, Dill CA. Constructs assessed by the GARS-2: factor analysis of data from the standardization sample. J Autism Dev Disord 2010;40(9):1118–30.

[30] Scott FJ, Baron-Cohen S, Bolton P, Brayne C. The CAST (childhood Asperger syndrome test): Preliminary development of a UK screen for mainstream primary-school-age children. Autism 2002;6(1):9–31.

[31] Pearson Education Ltd. Qualification codes. URL: https://www.pearsonclinical.co.uk/information/qualificationcodes.aspx.

[32] Kern JK, Geier DA, King PG, Sykes LK, Mehta JA, Geier MR. Shared brain connectivity issues, symptoms, and comorbidities in autism spectrum disorder, attention deficit/hyperactivity disorder, and Tourette syndrome. Brain Connect 2015;5(6):321–35.

[33] Kerns CM, Kendall PC. Autism and anxiety: overlap, similarities, and differences. In: Davis III TE, White SW, Ollendick TH, eds. Handbook of autism and anxiety. Cham: Springer, 2014:75–89.

[34] Mendle J, Beltz AM, Carter R, Dorn LD. Understanding puberty and its measurement: ideas for research in a new generation. J Res Adolesc 2019;29(1):82–95.

[35] Richardson H, Lisandrelli G, Riobueno-Naylor A, Saxe R. Development of the social brain from age three to twelve years. Nat Commun 2018;9(1):1027.

[36] Nelson EE, Jarcho JM, Guyer AE. Social re-orientation and brain development: an expanded and updated view. Dev Cogn Neurosci 2016;17:118–27.

[37] Patton JM, Cheng Y, Hong M, Diao Q. Detection and treatment of careless responses to improve item parameter estimation. J Educ Behav Stat 2019;44(3):309–41.

[38] Zablotsky B, Black LI, Maenner MJ, Schieve LA, Danielson ML, Bitsko RH, et al. Prevalence and trends of developmental disabilities among children in the United States: 2009–2017. Pediatrics 2019;144(4):e20190811.

[39] Glascoe FP. Screening for developmental and behavioral problems. Ment Retard Dev Disabil Res Rev 2005;11(3):173–9.

[40] Grzadzinski R, Dick C, Lord C, Bishop S. Parent-reported and clinician-observed autism spectrum disorder (ASD) symptoms in children with attention deficit/hyperactivity disorder (ADHD): implications for practice under DSM-5. Mol Autism 2016;7(1):7.

In: Building Children and Youth for the Future ISBN: 978-1-53618-806-6
Editors: Joav Merrick et al.

Chapter 9

THE DIGITIZATION OF SOCIETY AND ITS CHALLENGES TO CHILD DEVELOPMENT

Valentina Milenkova*, PhD and Boris Manov, PhD
Department of Sociology, South-West University "Neofit Rilski", Blagoevgrad, Bulgaria

ABSTRACT

In this chapter we aim to analyze some changes that occur in the child development and upbringing processes when entering the digital devices, like computers, tablets, Internet, mobile phones in the modern environment. The analysis focuses on the danger for children and the young generation of network dependence, online communication and digitization. How the parents control access to various digital devices? When they impose certain restrictions on the viewing of TV programs or usage of the Internet; and not only on what to watch, but as to how long. Do parents believe that the children could be protected from a variety of negative effects associated with aggression, high anxiety, uncertainty and emotional discomfort related to digital media. The paper is based on results obtained through qualitative methods in the course of research

* *Correspondence:* Professor Valentina Milenkova, PhD, Head, Department of Sociology, South-West University "Neofit Rilski", Blagoevgrad, Bulgaria. Email: vmilenkova@swu.bg.

project “Digital media literacy in the context of "knowledge society": State and challenges” H25/4, funded by National Science Fund, carried out in different Bulgarian regions. The main methods for obtaining information are In-Depth Interviews (30) and Focus group (5) with parents and representatives from different social groups and institutions.

INTRODUCTION

Digitization is a significant foundation of the modern knowledge society, operating in compacted spaces and times, in conditions of high mobility, in thc intcrchangeability of many tools and resources, as well as in the saturation of information sources and opportunities for influence. The knowledge society is a comprehensive and sustainable digitized and increasingly digital literacy becomes a condition for prosperity in the new realms of mobility and relationships.

At the same time, along with the positive aspects of digitization, there are a number of its negative effects, especially related to childhood development and the psyche. Digitization hides negative aspects related to the reduction of communication between people, enhancing privacy and closing of individuals, cyber threats, etc. This paper analyzes some changes that occur in the family upbringing processes when entering the digital devices, like: computers, tablets, Internet, mobile phones in the modern environment. How the parents control access to various digital devices? Do parents believe that the children could be protected from a variety of negative effects associated with aggression, high anxiety, uncertainty and emotional discomfort related to digital media socialization. The analysis focuses on the support that the children receive from parents in the context of mass digitization. Parents are the ones with whom children can discuss different topics, events, shows or movies viewed in the media as well as issues requiring further information or clarification from the parents.

The new environment requires the development of digital skills that enable effective information management and the proper use of ICT (1, 2).

Digitization, interactivity and virtuality are constantly opening up new possibilities and extending the boundaries of learning (3, 4).

Digital technologies have already changed the world, they have great potential to broaden the range of information they are handling, so they constantly adapt and become an integral part of the lives of modern people. The internet and new technologies create prerequisites being part of the global network, linked to the upgrading and dynamic flow of information, fast communication and easy access to various institutions. Digital media connect people to various social environments. Connected children and young people express their views through blogs, videos, social media, cartoons, hashtags, podcasts and other forms. They recognize the potential of digital resources to help them access information and seek solutions to problems affecting their communities (5).

Young people (aged 7-16 years) are the most closely related age group. Globally, 71% of them are online, compared to 48% (online) of the total population. Digital technologies provide opportunities for training and education for children. They also allow children to access information on issues that affect their communities and can provide them with a role to play in solving them.

OUR STUDY

The methodology that provides empirical material of this article includes qualitative methods: interviews and focus groups carried out under the project: "Digital media literacy in the context of "knowledge society": State and challenges" with team leader Valantina Milenkova. The fieldwork was conducted between March and May 2019 in different settlements of Southwest Bulgaria randomly selected.

The choice of methods followed the understanding that qualitative methods allow a deeper rationalizing different issues and a free sharing of views by respondents on the topics discussed. A total of 30 in depth interviews with university and school lecturers, researchers from scientific organizations, representatives of the non-government sector, politics, parents were held, following the methodological requirements laid down in the project.

The idea was to ask people from different social groups and institutions to share their understanding of digitization and digital literacy as well as the penetrating threat of using digital devices by children from different ages and in various educational contexts. The other method used was focus groups. There were carried out 5 focus groups with parents. The topics that were discussed in the group discussions included: benefits and damages from the digitalization of society; the dangers that can accompany web browsing, how children should use digital media, what role the family plays in the process of accessing digital media, what is the role of school and education in the process of digitization.

FINDINGS

During childhood, parents are the most important intermediaries in digital media socialization. Parents are the individuals who can provide the necessary cognitive and emotional balance to their children and in the later ages. Parents are aware of the serious challenges they face in the current situation related to various negative aspects of the action and content of digital media. Parents said that with age and school attendance, it is becoming increasingly difficult to control children's choice. The role of the school environment in this case is also of great importance. The assessment is that digital devices create conditions for widening divisions and inequalities among children, which complicates childhood assessments and perceptions. The basic element of digital socialization are the parents, the extent to which media messages break through the prism of group norms and rules in the relationship between the personality and society.

The family is of great importance to media socialization, because parents are the ones from whom the children learn various aspects of the world, including the media; kids are informed for different sources of information thanks to their parents, and they receive access to various digital devices: computers, tablets, Internet, mobile phones. Namely parents are the people who may impose certain restrictions on the viewing of TV programs or usage of the Internet; and not only on what to watch, but as to how long (6). Thus, the children can be protected from a variety of negative effects associated with aggression, high anxiety, uncertainty and emotional discomfort related with them. Parents are the ones with whom children can discuss a character, an event, a show or a movie viewed in the media as well as issues requiring further clarification, information or support from the parents.

Children get their first internet device at about 2 years of age - these are usually the smartphones that mothers give to children to have fun, not to cry and have fun on their own. More than half of Bulgarian households have tablets and just as much have smartphones.

For many children, the virtual world is more real than the real world. We all know how dangerous it can be surfing the net for a child that is 10 years old. Dangers and dating sites are also dangerous, where adolescents can be spoken by inappropriate people. There are various studies showing the impact of media usage on individuals, like violence and aggressive behavior in society (7). The role of the environment is also determined as a decisive factor (8). The Internet offers many opportunities but also hides a number of dangers, especially for those who do not know how to guarantee their security. Children are one of the most vulnerable groups. According to statistics, 50% of adolescents are already using the Internet before they reach 7 years. They often start communicating with different people across the screen, and this is an ideal opportunity for pedophiles and fraudsters.

The "National Safer Internet Center Marketlinx" conducted in 2016 a national representative survey on online behavior of children in Bulgaria (9). The study is concerned with exploring the use of the Internet, information and communication technologies by children between 9 and 17 years of age and their parents. The results showed that today's children are using the Internet ever earlier, more often and using increasingly diverse mobile devices, which increases the risks they face online. Bulgarian children on average start using the Internet at the age of eight, which is one year earlier than in 2010. They most often enter the online world for the first time in about 7 years. Around 97% are active users, a big leap compared to 81% in 2010. In addition, Bulgarian children go online more often in both school and non-academic days. Increased use increases the risks. 40% of children users have public Facebook profiles. The most endangered by the traps that the net hides are children aged 8-14 years.

Bulgarian children are increasingly falling on harmful content on the Internet. About 15% of them say they have been worried or afraid of something they've seen online in the past year. An alarmingly high percentage of social networking accounts are public, with the percentage being highest for an average age group (12-14). About 87% of children use social networks, which is significantly above 54% in 2010. One third of Bulgarian children has communicated with a person they have not met live. Online and offline child abuse has grown significantly over the past six years. About 30% have been offended or affected by a peer in the past year. The percentage of children using sexting (sending and receiving textual or visual content of a sexual nature) has not increased compared to 2010 (last survey), but remains worryingly high. (9).

Risks taking behavior hiding even innocent posting photos on the net that are not appropriate content can lead to harassment and extortion. Experts suggest that one of the most important factors to ensure the safety of children on the internet is to build a strong relationship of trust.

In the focus groups conducted in the author's survey in 2019 respondents shared that:

> "Parents must have constant control over what access children have to the Internet. Many people say today's children are born to be literate on the net. But, doing well does not make them digitally literate and does not make them safe for all risks online." (female, 45)

Parents commented that more than half of children get information on sites with inappropriate content, and they do not want it, which is very damaging to them.

> "Parents do not even suspect that children often go to inappropriate games - violent ones." (female, 35)

The age of admission of minors on the web, including making a social networking account, is steadily decreasing. Therefore, these activities should be under the control of parents.

> "Virtual communication itself can become aggression in real life." (male, 52)

Efforts are needed to protect children from the dangers of the Internet. The technique is constantly improving and more and more opportunities for Internet access appear. Progress in the field of technology places children with both unique opportunities and unpredictable dangers. One such danger is cyberbullying, which is a consequence of the uncritical manipulation of digital means. It consists in spreading discrediting information, photos, sending threatening messages, hacking into accounts and send messages to the contacts list in order defamation. The most important feature of online bullying is that it is public and destroys authority, and can negatively affect the confidence and self-concept of the child itself, since once shared information can spread very quickly across all platforms.

In one of the interviews, a parent said that after consulting with a psychologist he had his child close down his account to stop the attacks on him. Parents are concerned about the effect of the online world on the emotional and physical condition of their children. Children's threats online are equally real with adults, such as viruses, identity theft, online fraud. The problem is that children are more trustworthy and have less experience. Children can give information without thinking about the consequences that this may have.

Therefore, it is necessary to keep in touch with the children in order to be reasonable and to use the Internet responsibly, to be aware of the dangers in the network. Thus, the Internet will be a useful means of communicating and obtaining information that will not threaten their security.

Parents in focus groups say that in order to protect their children they must have basic knowledge of the Internet and what their children do when they communicate by instant messaging or "chat," browse web pages or do something else on the web. This information can be obtained through a variety of software programs that offer parental control, which stops inappropriate messages and images that appear on the computer screen, and prevents children from opening dangerous pages. It was shared that:

> "These filtering or blocking programs do not provide 100 percent protection. Additionally, older youngsters understand computers and learn how to ignore or outsmart these programs." (male, 43)

That is why parents have to determine when children can use the Internet and for how long, as well as what websites they can visit and what websites are forbidden. According to parents, this should not have the nature of a ban or coercion, but of explanation and discussion with the children, and why it is necessary. One of the participants in the focus groups said that "children should go to specific educational sites dedicated to animals, nature, science" (female, 38). Or "make a list of Internet libraries, dictionaries and tutorials" (female, 40).

Another problem that parents have pointed out is that they cannot keep track of what their children do when they are not at home. It is therefore important that the control of the internet is not a single action, and it is a continuous process of mutual trust, the formation of values, the observance of rules so that kids can make the right decisions even when they are alone. In this sense, the finding that the protection, which parents can ensure by monitoring children's activities, is limited. The principles that parents teach their children and the example they give can achieve much more in this respect. Therefore, it is time to discuss with children the dangers of using the Internet.

> "Open communication with children is the best protection against hidden threats on the Internet." (male, 46)

There are a variety of digital devices, each of which is associated with different benefits:

Mobile phones

In a survey conducted with individuals aged 18-65 years (9), about 75% of respondents said the average age at which children receive their first smartphone is 10 years. The smartphone provides a number of advantages with regard to the constant connection and location of the children: where they are, what friends they are with, when they are coming back, as well as to stay in contact for an extended period of time or to have a quick response if parents need to respond quickly when needed. The advantages of smartphones, however, can also become their shortcomings because they are personal devices and may not always have full control over them by parents, and that makes children highly vulnerable. In the focus groups, some of the parents shared how they could limit the continued use of smartphones:

> "I basically strive to give myself a personal example by not keeping my phone on the table, not calling while driving; I try to show that you do not have to have a phone in hand and follow the flow of events." (female, 50)

> "I think there should be limitations, for example, how many hours a day the phone can use, but I think this is difficult to realize, and it is known that when you restrict someone, you stimulate him to show a trick, to try to invent ways to disregard the restrictions, so great care must be taken." (male, 45)

Online games

Massively children aged 3 to 17 years play video and online games. Children can play alone or with some of their peers they know, or with others who do not know it but have met online. The games form different skills related to rapid reaction, imagination and creativity, perspective thinking, teamwork. Some of the games also have a cognitive element. Online gaming is a prerequisite for creating new contacts with other gamers, even from around the world, which opens the possibility of abuse.

Threats related to online gaming can be manifested in several ways:

- Violence is present in the games, quality of vengeance is developing; the very process of play is accompanied by nervous overload, high adrenaline, which affects the child's psyche
- The games go through different levels, which requircs a prolonged stay in front of the computer and actually tears the child out of his or her schooling or homework duties. Children do not exercise and do little to do.
- Children can create relationships with other players and become subject to online harassment.

In the focus groups, parents say that they are trying to discuss their children's online games in order to give them advice or to share their personal experiences, to help their children, to support them when they have difficulty.

Social networks

Teens are the most active age group on social networks, using more than one platform but spending at least 3-4 hours daily. Moreover, it is the contacts they make on social networks that are a priority for them, rather than finding the learning materials they need for school or university. Social networks become very important because they contribute to developing age identity, peer association, posting information about different events or people. In this sense, social networks develop dependence on teenagers as they are the basis of contacts with strangers, sharing inappropriate content, or cyberbullying. It is therefore necessary to set boundaries with regard to the long standing in the social networks and the risks that it hides.

In the focus groups, parents share that one of the ways of control is to regulate privacy settings, and to monitor the child's online activities, which would allow parents to respond preventively. According to our respondents, profiling and social networking should be limited as long as possible to protect children from adverse and risky influences or addictions.

The school

The school is a key institution for the development of digital skills, through the teaching methods it applies, as well as the educational approaches and ways of interaction that it carries out in its work. Based on teaching methods, teachers can stimulate teamwork, interactivity, critical thinking, and it is these skills that underpin the comprehension of information and how to counter cyberbullying and the various risks associated with digitization. One of the main problems of modern education is that it does not develop young people's thinking and reflexivity, which is why they trust the information on the Internet, trust the strangers unconditionally and seek their approval. Therefore, school and education in general need to be able to form the access skill to a large amount of information, which creates a need for management, integration and evaluation skills.

Modern education stimulates the development of critical thinking; there is a series of examples in this direction that are indicative of the fact that approach to digital technologies are entering and changing the existing methods of education and teaching in educational institutions. Actions to implement digital technologies in education are adopted:

- investments in the purchase of digital equipment and the creation of laboratories and cabinets in schools and universities;
- creating computer programs for learning purposes;

- inclusion of information technology classes in schools' curricula;
- conducting projects and scientific forums on the issues of digitalization of education.

The main goal of educational technologies is to improve not only the learning process but also the efficiency of the education system (10). In the foundation of modern educational technologies is laid the integration of information and communication tools and achievements. What integrates digital technologies is enhanced interactivity, based on the concepts of cooperative learning, collaborative learning, e-learning, for the achievement of digital literacy (11). A basic feature of these processes and mobile learning as a whole is the desire to achieve a kind of an autonomy of the individual student/pupil (12). That is why the attention of specialists focuses on the theories of learning and their application in the teaching of various subjects (13). The following approaches are implemented in education:

- Learning in experience and through experience. What characterizes the educational technologies in the foundation of which underlies learning through experience and in experience is the creation of life-related situations. In this type of learning problems, which are close to the real life ones have an important place. Professionals talk about so-called authentic problems. Their solution allows them to create an educational environment in which the traditional roles of the teacher and the pupils change. Pupils master the material as role-playing activities, where they improve their socio-cultural competencies (to fulfil certain social roles in a particular socio-cultural context). This type of learning offers opportunities to use preliminary knowledge.
- Problem-based learning is related to solving cognitive problems. In organizing it, the model of scientific knowledge follows, it is realized through the following stages:

- Identifying the general subject by the teacher, but it can also be formulated by the pupils. Its importance and relevance is important for the pupils involved in the research.
- Decomposing the general topic of micro-topics and each group chooses their micro topic to work. This can be done through brainstorming and a through a conceptual network (the key words and logical links between them.
- Planning and implementing the research process.
- Data collection and preparation of a report on the activity carried out.
- Presentation of the development through a computer presentation.
- Assessment of the presentation of each group of the other participants. Criteria discussed in advance are used, and they accepted by all participants.
- Global-oriented learning is a conception based on inter-subject relations. The cross-border nature of cognitive activities carried out by pupils is a favorable prerequisite for improving their socio-cultural competences as well as the use of knowledge acquired on different subjects and aimed at achieving a higher level of education.

DISCUSSION

Digitization is valued as an important process that has actively penetrated society by changing all areas of political, professional, social life and personal relationships and activities of people. Digitization also has negative impacts and effects associated with: diminishing social skills, long hours spent at the computer, little time for school activities. Many of the online activities - such as online games - are related to violence, nervous tension and stress. Moreover, inclusion in social networks lies threats from contact with strangers and cyberbullying. All this is a consequence of the fragile age in which children encounter digital devices and lack social experience and skills. In this context, it is necessary for parents to be with their children, to communicate with them, to exchange information about both the events at school and the people they meet online. The experience of the parents themselves and the example they give to their children is very important. Another significant actor in countering digital risks is the school. The contribution of teachers in this direction is expressed in the application of different teaching methods in which the group work, individual participation and thinking, the ability to reason children are activated. It is through stimulating social contacts based on shared learning and research, as well as stimulating the reflexivity of children, that ways of dealing with many of the risks of digitization can be outlined. The good connection between parents and school is the basis for protecting children from the negative effects of digitization and developing skills for critical thinking, sociality, personal activity and civic behavior.

The threats of digitization are to deepen social divisions, to strengthen the opposition between communities and individuals, to social exclusion of large groups of people who lack the resources and potential to follow digital changes and their innovative states.

More systematic action is needed, longer-term vision, more focused strategies on how to develop personal and social skills of individuals. Bulgarian education is not always able to meet the new requirements and to take effective account of changes. In this sense, complicating the responsibilities, the work and the nature of the obligations becomes a prerequisite for the formation of the population.

ACKNOWLEDGMENTS

The article has been developed in the framework of the research project "Digital media literacy in the context of "knowledge society": State and challenges" № КП–06–Н25/4, funded by National Science Fund – Bulgaria.

REFERENCES

[1] Milenkova V, Keranova D, Peicheva D. Digital skills and new media and information literacy as a conditions of cigitization. Appl Hum Factors Ergonomics 2020:65-72.

[2] Cartelli A, Fostering 21st century digital literacy and technical competency. Hershey, PA: IGI Global, 2013.

[3] Rosengren KE. Media effects and beyond: Culture, socialization and lifestyles. London, UK: Routledge, 2014.

[4] Henriksen C, Media and ICT in a learning perspective. URL: http://www.dpu.dk/ en/research/ researchprogrammes mediaandict/.

[5] Adeyemon E. Integrating digital literacies into outreach services for underserved youth populations. Reference Librarian 2009;50(1):85-98.

[6] Greenfield P, Yan Z, Children, adolescents, and the internet: A new field of inquiry in developmental psychology. Dev Psychol 2006;42(3):391-4.

[7] Lemish D. Children and media. A global perspective. Oxford, UK: Wiley Blackwell, 2015.

[8] Anderson JA. The production of media violence and aggression research. A cultural analysis. Am Behav Scientist 2008;51(8):1260-79.

[9] National representative survey on online behavior of children in Bulgaria, carried out by National Safer Internet Center Marketlinx, 2016. URL: https://www.unicef.bg/ assets/NewsPics/2017/PDFs/BulgarianNationaResearch2016_Summary_BG.pdf.

[10] Krumsvik R. Situated learning and teachers' digital competence. Educ Inform Technol 2008;13(4):279-90.

[11] Punie Y. Learning spaces: An ICT-enabled model of future learning in the knowledge-based society. Eur J Educ 2007;42:185–99.

[12] Sefton-Green J, Nixon H, Erstad O. Reviewing approaches and perspectives on "digital literacy". Pedagogies 2009;4(2):107-25.

[13] Eshet-Alkalai Y, Chajut E. Changes over time in digital literacy. Cyber Psychol Behav 2009;12(6):713-5.

In: Building Children and Youth for the Future ISBN: 978-1-53618-806-6
Editors: Joav Merrick et al.

Chapter 10

HOSPITAL EXPERIENCE USING CULTURAL INTERPRETERS WITH THE ORTHODOX JEWISH COMMUNITY

Vincent J Palusci*[*]*, MD, MS, Israel Rosman, MBA, Michelle Romano Shami, MS, LCSW and Dennis Sklenar, LCSW

New York University Langone Health and New York University Grossman School of Medicine, New York, United States of America

ABSTRACT

The Orthodox Jewish Community has religious and cultural traditions that separate it from mainstream society and that impact the medical evaluation and reporting of suspected child maltreatment. We designed and implemented a program of cultural interpreters in two hospitals in 2015 to improve communication with this community for better identification and mandated reporting. Children from the Orthodox Jewish Community at two hospitals were referred to our child protection committee. We reviewed case logs and social work notes during 2016-2019 and noted membership in the Orthodox Jewish Community, child

[*] Corresponding Author's Email: Vincent.palusci@nyulangone.org.

gender, age, concerns of specific abuse types, whether the case was reported to child protective services, whether the program was used, and family and staff reactions. The proportion of reported cases of suspected child neglect initially declined while there was no change in mandated abuse reporting. These changes did not persist through 2019, and fewer than one fourth of eligible families were documented as having received the program. In the cases with program documentation, staff expressed satisfaction in obtaining more complete medical history from Orthodox families when evaluating suspected child maltreatment, and families appreciated the interest and support. We concluded that cultural interpreters are useful for obtaining information in hospitals for cases of suspected child abuse and neglect, but additional staff training is needed to improve implementation and further study is needed to determine if cultural interpreters can reliably improve child maltreatment reporting outcomes.

INTRODUCTION

The Orthodox Jewish Community (OJC) has religious and cultural traditions that separate it from mainstream society and impact the medical evaluation and reporting of suspected child maltreatment (CM). The OJC is composed of numerous groups such as the Hasidim, which differ from the "modern" orthodox community that incorporates secular culture, and the OJC has separate religious, cultural, and education systems (1, 2). Fertility rates for OJC families are more than double that of the general population (3), and the number of families and the number of children in those families is growing. Members of the OJC generally do not watch commercial television, listen to radio, or read materials in the popular press. Groups within the OJC look to their community's leaders for guidance and information, and it is believed that members of OJC generally do not receive injury prevention or other public health messages, although this information is increasingly being distributed at the direction of their community leaders (4).

The OJC's isolation affects medical care in a number of ways, including the mandatory reporting of suspected CM. There have been infection outbreaks (5-7) and injuries related to their practices (5, 8-10). For example, a review noted three important factors that contribute to child sexual abuse in the OJC: the perceived authority of religious leaders that allows them to operate without challenge or accountability; religious doctrine that elevates traditional religious practice, patriarchy and self-governance over effective policies to protect children; and a repressive attitude towards sexuality and sexual education (11).

Historically, reported neglect is more common than abuse in U.S., and an important number of child injuries are the result of physical neglect or inadequate supervision (12). Large families with many children have increased risk for injury resulting from inadequate supervision (13). In the US, all states have some form of mandated reporting of suspected CM (14), and medical providers are an important source of CM reports (12). Children of the OJC may then be less likely to be reported for suspected CM if they are directed away from emergency departments to private practitioners who are part of their community (15).

When they do seek care outside the OJC, privacy concerns and fear of government involvement can lead OJC members not to reveal to medical staff how an accidental injury occurred, creating misunderstandings that can sometimes engender antagonism and frustration among both families and mandated reporters (16). Difficulties can also arise because of their fear of spreading *leshon ha-ra* (derogatory speech about another person) or *mesira* (informing on Jews to secular authorities) (17). While strong networks and social systems are protective factors at higher ecological levels, cultural practices such as refusal to share personal or family information to those perceived to be outside the community can hinder the medical evaluation of potential CM. Suspicions of CM may arise when incomplete or no medical history information is presented, for example, to explain how an injury occurred (18).

A number of improvements in practice have been proposed across disciplines, and a broad social work approach has been piloted in Israel to address society-level risk factors for abuse (19, 20). To address cultural issues in health care specifically, cultural competence has gained attention from health care policy-makers, providers, and insurers as a strategy to improve quality and eliminate racial/ethnic disparities (21). The goal of cultural competence is to create a health care system and workforce that are capable of delivering the highest quality care to every patient regardless of race, ethnicity, culture, or language proficiency. Integrated models of care and safety have been proposed for use in hospital settings, including multidisciplinary child protection teams (16, 22, 23). Given these concerns, a goal for a culturally competent medical program should be to avoid cultural obstacles that may lead to under- or over-reporting of child abuse and neglect, the consequences of which have been noted (24).

Our institution encompasses hospitals, clinics and physicians' offices in the NY metropolitan area where young children are assessed for potentially abusive or neglectful injuries. Within a 75-mile radius, there are a mixture of OJC sects in networks extending from upstate New York to Long Island and to Lakewood, New Jersey, and it has been estimated that at least 500,000 of New York City's 8.5 million population are part of the OJC and live in well-defined geographic areas (25). Starting in 2013, our patient liaison department and child protection committee began to consider a cultural competence model as the basis for a program to improve the care of OJC children with suspected abuse and neglect. We first looked at one model that has been described for use in an ultra-orthodox community in Israel (the *Haredi*) to address the group's specific internal language and cultural codes (26).

Realizing that a response which went beyond language was needed, we implemented a program of "cultural interpreters" (CIs) in 2015 in two hospitals. Staff can contact these CIs when they have concerns about child maltreatment among the OJC. This program was designed to build upon already strong language interpretation services by adding trained members of the OJC who could 'translate' the information that was needed and better explain our services and responsibilities in a sensitive way that would be better understood and accepted by OJC families. In a preliminary assessment, we found a total of 38 cases, including 18 from 2011 before implementation and 20 from 2016 (27). Among cases referred to the hospital child protection committee, fewer (one-fourth) were reported to child protective services after cultural interpreters were implemented than were before (one-third). There were fewer cases of neglect referred to our committee (11/18 in 2011 vs. 9/20 in 2016) and fewer neglect reports (4/11 vs. 1/9) after implementation. The number of abuse cases rose as did the proportion that was reported. Overall, nearly two-thirds (25/38) of committee referrals were boys, and most (29/38) were younger than 5 years old. After implementation, the proportion of boys being reported decreased (4/11 vs. 3/14), and a greater decrease in reporting was noted among younger children. While we concluded that our program of cultural interpreters had some impact on the number of children being referred and reported for suspected neglect, there were some limitations including the small number of cases available for analysis and the lack of information about maltreatment concern and injury type.

In the current study, we sought to extend our understanding of best practices for responding to concerns about child maltreatment in the OJC by reviewing additional cases in our CI program with comparisons assessing use of the program and reporting rates by type of abuse. We hypothesized that there were continued declines in neglect reporting rates with little or no differences in reporting for abuse.

OUR STUDY

The hospital child protection committee is composed of physicians, nurses, social workers, and other hospital professionals who assist staff at both hospitals in reporting procedures, track patient outcomes, conduct quality assurance activities, and provide education and training for staff about child abuse and neglect in a model used by other children's hospital-based teams (28). Committee members may assist clinical staff, consult directly with families, and make recommendations about CM reporting, but staff are not required to follow these recommendations.

We implemented internal procedures as part of this pilot project in 2015 as part of our quality improvement efforts to improve care for the OJC population. Using a framework that goes beyond the language interpretation services regulatorily required in healthcare facilities (29), our child protection committee and patient liaison program identified "cultural interpreters" (CIs) among our patient advocate staff to facilitate culturally competent communication with OJC families. These interpreters are hospital staff who function in the medical center as patient liaisons and advocates who are actual or perceived members of the OJC. Different from the "cultural elder," "cultural wayfinder," or "speaking Haredi" models, these interpreters do not treat or direct families in how or where to seek care; rather, they explain medical and hospital procedures and CM mandated reporting, and they reassure the family that information being provided about the injury, family members, and home environment is the standard of care needed to evaluate the child's medical condition. When the hospital child protection committee is notified about a child with concerns of CM, the cultural interpreter is contacted to assist the family by providing needed information and helping their understanding of medical procedures. They are available in-person or by telephone, which is especially valuable during late evening or early morning hours. They also advise staff on best practices for interacting with OJC families. On-call social workers and child abuse pediatricians who have training and experience to understand these cultural issues are also contacted and can assist in CM reporting procedures.

Study design and analysis

In order to assess whether there were any changes in CM reporting after implementation, we conducted a retrospective review of administrative records from years 2017-2019 as a convenience sample with families who self-identified as being from the OJC to augment previously collected data for 2011 and 2016. Social work notes were also reviewed to identify documentation of the intervention and family reaction. For this analysis, the child's age, gender, injury, primary maltreatment concern, and whether the case was reported to child protective services by our institution were collected, including outcomes of the report (report accepted, report not accepted, not reported-case already open, or not reported-ruled out). Rates for reporting were analyzed by child age, gender and CM type. Trends were assessed by year before and after the intervention, initially using an intention to treat design. Chi-squared and Fisher's exact tests were used as appropriate to parametrically compare proportions, with $p < 0.05$ taken as statistically significant. Abuse was defined to include physical, sexual and psychological abuse, while neglect included physical and medical neglect. In other analyses, individual CM types were assessed. Minutes from child protection meetings for the applicable periods were reviewed, and committee comments and staff and family reactions were noted. Additional analyses were conducted in which characteristics for cases with documented use of the intervention were compared to those without such documentation available. This study was reviewed and deemed exempt from further review by our institutional research committee.

FINDINGS

A total of 92 cases meeting inclusion criteria were found, including 18 in 2011 before implementation, and 74 after, with an overall decline in OJC cases referred to our hospital child protection committee over time (see Table 1). Almost half (45%) were reported to child protective services after program of cultural interpreters was implemented, compared to one-third before, reflecting an increased reporting proportion over time. There were fewer cases of neglect referred to our committee (11/18 in 2011) compared to 39/74 after implementation. The number of abuse cases did not change, but the proportion that was reported increased (29% before, 51% after). Overall, more than half of committee referrals were boys, and almost two-thirds were younger than 5 years old. There was no important change in the proportion of boys being reported, but a small increase in reporting was noted among younger children (0-4y). Most abuse concerns related to physical abuse, and most neglect related to general physical neglect. Later years showed decreases in abuse reporting and increases in reported neglect (see Figure 1). None of the differences in proportions were statistically significant.

Meeting minutes noted that committee members reported that families expressed better understanding of medical procedures and legal mandates for professionals caring for their children after implementation. Medical providers expressed more satisfaction after being able to make more complete and accurate reports when indicated. There was documentation in case records of the intervention being used in just more than 20% of eligible OJC cases during 2016-2019 (15/74) (see Table 1). The intervention was documented as being used more frequently among older children (5y or older), females, and when there were concerns of neglect (see Table 2). The overall proportion of reported neglect cases rose during 2016-2019 (see figure 1). Initially, the overall reported proportion declined, then rose, then fell again, and the proportion reported was not significantly different between those with and without documentation of the intervention (47% v. 44%, $p > 0.05$). Small numbers with limited statistical power prevented meaningful comparison of varying maltreatment types or reporting outcomes.

Table 1. Comparison of child and report factors over time in all cases

	2011	**2016**	**2017**	**2018**	**2019**	**Totals**
Total Cases	**18**	**20**	**27**	**14**	**13**	**92**
Age						
0-4y	13	13	19	6	7	58
5 or older	5	7	8	8	6	34
Gender						
Female	7	6	13	6	8	40
Male	11	14	14	8	5	52
Maltreatment						
Abuse:	7	11	11	7	6	42
Physical Abuse	7	9	11	6	6	39
Sexual Abuse	0	2	0	1	0	3
Neglect:	11	9	16	7	7	50
Physical Neglect	8	4	12	6	5	35
Medical Neglect	3	5	4	1	2	15
Report Status						
Reported:	6	5	14	7	7	39
Accepted	6	5	14	6	6	37
Not Accepted	0	0	0	1	1	2
Not Reported:	12	15	13	7	6	53
Open Case	2	4	4	2	2	14
Ruled Out	10	11	9	5	4	39
CI Documented, %	0	10	30	21	15	20

CI = Cultural Interpreter.

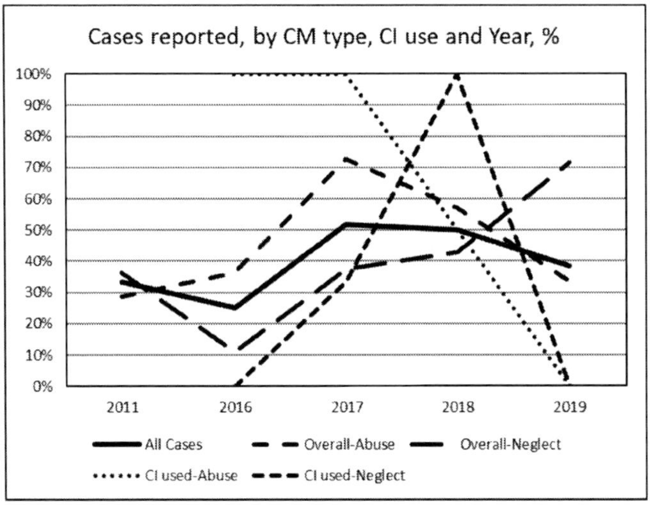

Figure 1.

Table 2. Comparison of child and report factors in cases, 2016-2019, by CI documentation

	Documented	%	Not Documented	%	Totals
2016-2019	**15**	**100**	**59**	**100**	**74**
Age					
0-4y	6	40	39	66	45
5 or older	9	60	20	34	29
Gender					
Female	7	47	26	44	33
Male	8	53	33	56	41
Maltreatment					
Abuse:	6	40	29	49	35
Physical Abuse	6		26		32
Sexual Abuse	0		3		3
Neglect:	9	60	30	51	39
Physical Neglect	6		21		27
Medical Neglect	3		9		12
Report Status					
Reported:	7	47	26	44	33
Accepted	6		25		31
Not Accepted	1		1		2
Not Reported:	8	53	33	56	41
Open Case	1		11		12
Ruled Out	7		22		29

CI = Cultural Interpreter.

Discussion

Our preliminary experience with the use of "cultural interpreters" was promising, but over time, the number of cases with documentation of their use declined and the reporting proportions increased. Not all CM reports can be avoided, and reports have continued to be made when indicated but with more complete medical history available to facilitate investigation and provide services. The non-significant differences in patient age, gender, CM type and reporting appear to reflect what happens in cases at our institution overall. The documented use of cultural interpreters in neglect cases by our hospital child protection committee supports our assumption that reports for suspected neglect may be associated with inadequate medical information obtained from OJC families. This has been shown to differ from abuse, which, in the case of sexual abuse, seems to be derived more from religious authority and tradition rather than from the need for cultural interpretation and communication in the hospital (11, 30).

It is unclear to us why fewer than one fourth of families who could potentially benefit from cultural interpreters were documented to have been provided the intervention. There did not appear to be differential application based on child gender or age, but they were used more with concerns of neglect. We have noted that when these procedures could not be used, parents and staff often expressed frustration or anger about CM reporting and outcomes. We speculate that they were not used because of staff unavailability, lack of staff knowledge on how to access them, or lack of knowledge about the program overall given staff turnover during the study period over time. In addition, it is possible that more OJC families were provided the intervention, but not documented in the medical record or were not referred to our committee. This misclassification could skew our results toward finding no differences between the study groups.

The overall proportion of cases reported to CPS by our hospital child protection committee, the relationship to specific CM type, and changes over time are not addressed by our study. Similar to national data, most of the children referred to our committee in this sample were young and therefore less able to disclose what had happened to them (12). We speculate that the higher proportion of boys may reflect cultural practices in the OJC in which boys are treated differently from girls by parents. One hospital trauma registry, for example, reported data for 697 pediatric trauma patients, of which 87 were reported as suspected abuse victims. This was 8% of their pediatric trauma patients with a median age of 6 months, ranging from newborn to age 10 years, and most victims (55%) were male (23). Another prospective multi-center study of 968 consecutive cases referred to child protection teams in six medical centers in Israel noted high rates of reporting (61.7%) among cases referred to their teams, with a child's young age and other family factors being associated with the decision to report (31). Differences in family class and ethnicity have also been shown to have effects on the identification and response to CM, and parents with high social status often resist the investigation (32).

We continue to believe the use of cultural interpreters can be helpful for our OJC patients, families and staff. While medical providers have traditional duties to maintain patient privacy and confidentiality, they are also required by state law to report suspected child abuse and neglect. Jewish law and scholarship recognize this potential *halakhic* problem that emerges if patient confidentiality must be broken because it is biblically mandated not to slander your neighbor (as included in Leviticus 19:16, Proverbs 25:9, and Psalms 34:14). Thus, while divulging confidential patient information can be considered grounds for professional negligence, it is noted to actually be obligatory by Jewish law when required for the safety of the patient and the public when child abuse is suspected (17, 33). CIs have the potential to navigate these concerns to the benefit of the child, family and staff.

LIMITATIONS

This was a single-institution study with a small number of subjects that limited its statistical power and generalizability. Given our location in a very large metropolitan area with multiple medical centers, the lack of pediatric trauma center designation during the study period, and selective use of our pediatric services by the OJC, we suspect that our experience is not comparable to that of other centers. The mix of cases and community resources may impact the functions our committee is asked to accomplish, and our population and child protection committee may be unique. One survey of child protection teams noted that experts believed that effective teams should provide communication of findings to appropriate agencies, court testimony, medical consultations, multidisciplinary case review, and forensic interviews (34). In our setting, communication, consultation and case review are considered primary functions, with less interviewing and court appearance needed. In addition, child sexual abuse has been reported in other Jewish communities, but we saw few cases at our institution (10). Thus it is unclear whether our program of cultural interpreters would have the similar results in other settings with a different mix of CM types.

There are also several limitations to procedures of this nature being used in a large, metropolitan area with diverse cultures. The OJC lives in multiple counties and states with different child protective services agencies and reporting practices. Language may be an issue, with some members of the OJC speaking only Hebrew or Yiddish. The OJC is not homogenous, and cultural interpreters, while actual members of or perceived as members of the OJC, are not necessarily part of all these individual sects. This has been noted to be perhaps the most daunting challenge facing professionals who work with Orthodox Jews (35). Safety concerns about other children in the home may not allow for any delay in reporting while the cultural interpreters are becoming involved and some health professionals choose to make reports irrespective of our committee procedures because of legal mandates. Lastly, while we aim to obtain the best information from families, individuals may still continue not to share information or obfuscate or obstruct an evaluation because of their perceived guilt or other reasons. Brofsky (17) has concluded that concerns about *mesira* and *leshon ha-ra,* however, should not stand in the way of taking proper actions to protect victims and prevent further abuse, and he has noted that there are *halakhic* sources which demand and obligate the medical community and the OJC to stop and prevent sexual, physical, and emotional abuse.

CONCLUSION

It appears that our program of cultural interpreters had some impact on families and the number of children being referred and reported at our institution, but the impact has decreased over time. It would be helpful to perform additional studies of the use of CIs, particularly with randomized, blinded designs. We hope to extend our understanding of best practices for responding to concerns about child maltreatment in the OJC by reviewing additional evidence-informed, culturally-relevant strategies that can be adapted from other communities. We also hope to improve our current strategy using staff education to increase referrals to our CI program. Feedback will continue to be sought from OJC representatives as well as directly from families receiving care at our institution. Our committee will continue to work with medical professionals and social workers to assure these procedures are used and to record their perceptions of the evaluation and reporting processes. This will inform further development and implementation of more effective medical care and compliance with mandated reporting laws for OJC families in our health care system.

ACKNOWLEDGMENTS

The authors would like to thank Thomas Sedgwick, MSW, ACSW for his help in designing and implementing the cultural interpreters program, and Beatrice Guanco and Sydney Tack for their assistance with record review. This paper was presented in part at the Challenged Child Conference at Hadassah Hospital in Jerusalem, Israel on December 2, 2019.

REFERENCES

[1] Schick M. A census of Jewish day schools in the United States 2008–2009. Avi Chai Foundation, 2009. URL: http://avichai.org/wp-content/uploads/2010/06/Census-of-JDS-in-the-US-2008-09-Final.pdf.

[2] Cooperman A, Smith GA. Eight facts about Orthodox Jews from the Pew Research Survey 2013. URL: http://www.pewresearch.org/fact-tank/2013/10/17/eight-facts-about-orthodox-jews-from-the-pew-research-survey/.

[3] Cohen SM, Ukeles JB, Miller R. Jewish Community Study of New York: 2011 comprehensive report. UJA-Federation of New York, Jewish Policy and Action Research 2012. URL: www.ujafedny.org/jewish-community-study-of-new-york-2011.

[4] Jewish Community Health Initiative. (n.d.). Helping Jews lead healthier lives. URL: http://jewhealth.org/.

[5] Blank S, Myers JE, Pathela P, Washburn K, Varma JK, Hadler JL, et al. Neonatal herpes simplex virus infection following Jewish ritual circumcision that included direct oral genital suction in New York City. MMWR 2012;61(22):405-9.

[6] Lighter-Fisher J, Phillips MS, Stachel A, Chopra A, Rosman I, Fisher, JC, et al., Geographic cluster of community-acquired methicillin-resistant Staphylococcus aureus infections among pediatric patients from Brooklyn, New York. Poster Abstracts OFID IDWeek 2016;1(Suppl 1):S1.

[7] Rosen JB, Arciuolo RJ, Khawja AM, Fu J, Giancotti FR, Zucker JR. Public health consequences of a 2013 measles outbreak in New York City. JAMA Pediatr 2018. doi:10.1001/jamapediatrics.2018.1024.

[8] Greenbaum AL. Vowing to face who we really are: Child abuse and domestic violence in the Jewish community. J Relig Abuse 2002;4(1):69-76.

[9] Shoufani A, Golan J. Shabbes burn, a burn that occurs solely among Jewish orthodox children due to accidental shower from overhead water heaters. Burns 2003;29:61-4.

[10] Rosmarin DH, Pirutinsky S, Appel M, Kaplan T, Pelcovitz D. Childhood sexual abuse, mental health, and religion across the Jewish community. Child Abuse Negl 2018;81:21-8.

[11] Mendes P, Pinskier M, McCurdy S, Averbukh R. Ultra-orthodox Jewish communities and child sexual abuse: A case study of the Australian Royal Commission and its implications for faith-based communities. Children Australia 2019. URL: https://doi.org/10.1017/cha.2019.44.

[12] Administration for Children and Families, Administration on Children, Youth and Families, Children's Bureau. Child Maltreatment 2018, Washington, DC: US Department of Health Human Services 2019. URL: https://www.acf.hhs.gov/cb/resource/child-maltreatment-2018.

[13] Hymel KP and the Committee on Child Abuse and Neglect. When is lack of supervision neglect? Pediatrics 2006;118(3):1296-8.

[14] Palusci VJ, Vandervort FE. Universal reporting laws and child maltreatment report rates in large U.S. counties. Child Youth Serv Rev 2014;38:20-8.

[15] Holter JC, Friedman SB. Child abuse: Early case finding in the emergency department. Pediatrics 1968;42:128-38.

[16] White S, Wastell D, Smith S, Hall C, Whitaker E, Debelle G, et al. Improving practice in safeguarding at the interface between hospital services and children's social care: A mixed-methods case study. Health Serv Deliv Res 2015;3(4). URL: https://www.ncbi.nlm.nih.gov/books/NBK274394/ doi: 10.3310/hsdr03040.

[17] Brofsky D. Discussing and reporting abuse – a Halakhic perspective. Tradition 2017;50(2):60-77.

[18] Christian CW and the Committee on Child Abuse and Neglect. The evaluation of suspected child physical abuse. Pediatrics 2015;135(5):e1337-54.

[19] Palusci VJ, Haney ML. Strategies to prevent child maltreatment and integration into practice. APSAC Adv 2010;22(1):8-17.

[20] Katz C, McLeigh J, Ben Arieh A. Reflections on the traditional role of social workers in child protection: Lessons learned from the Strong Communities Initiative in Israel. Int J Child Maltreat 2019;2:199–210.

[21] Betancourt JR, Green AR, Emilio Carrillo E, Park ER. Cultural competence and health care disparities: Key perspectives and trends. Health Aff 2005;24(2):499-505.

[22] Connolly S. Everyone's business: Developing an integrated model of care to respond to child abuse in a pediatric hospital setting. Soc Work Health Care 2012;51(1):36-52.

[23] Draus JM. A multidisciplinary child protection team improves care of non-accidental trauma patients. Am Surg 2017;83(May):477-81.

[24] Raz M. Unintended consequences of expanded mandatory reporting laws. Pediatrics 2017;139(2):e20163511.

[25] Gallagher P. Identification and analysis of Orthodox Jewish enclaves in Brooklyn, New York: A GIS based approach. Mid States Geog 2009;42:83-9.

[26] Band-Winterstein T, Freund A. Is it enough to 'Speak Haredi'? Cultural sensitivity in social workers encountering Jewish Ultra-Orthodox clients in Israel. British J Soc Work 2015;45:968–87.

[27] Palusci VJ, Sedgwick TW, Rosman I. Using cultural interpreters with the Orthodox Jewish Community. In: James-Brown C, Wolfe DS, Collins J, Adams R, eds. Child maltreatment in insular and isolated communities. Washington, DC: CWLA Press, 2018:81-93.

[28] National Association of Children's Hospitals and Related Institutions. Defining the children's hospital role in child maltreatment 2006. URL: http://bsfi.barnlakar foreningen.se/wp-content/uploads/sites/13/2016/03/nachri.full_.guidelines05.pdf.

[29] Reardon C. More than words — Cultural competency in healthcare. Soc Work Today 2009;9(3):12. URL: http://www.socialworktoday.com/archive/051109 p12.shtml.

[30] Palusci VJ, Vandervort FE, Lewis JM. Does changing mandated reporting laws improve child maltreatment reporting in large U.S. counties? Child Youth Serv Rev 2016;66:170-9.

[31] Benbenishty R, Jedwab M, Chen W, Glasser S, Slutzky H, Siegal G, et al. Predicting the decisions of hospital based child protection teams to report to child

protective services, police and community welfare services. Child Abuse Negl 2014;38:11–24.

[32] Aadnanes M. Social workers' challenges in the assessment of child abuse and maltreatment: Intersections of class and ethnicity in child protection cases. Crit Rad Soc Work 2017;5(3):335-50.

[33] Dollin Y, Roth J. Psychiatric malpractice in Jewish law. J Jewish Ethics 2018;4(1):47-94.

[34] Kistin CJ, Tien I, Bauchner H, Parker V, Leventhal JM. Factors that influence the effectiveness of child protection teams. Pediatrics 2010;126:94-100.

[35] Schnall E. Multicultural counseling and the Orthodox Jew. J Counsel Dev 2006;84:275-82.

In: Building Children and Youth for the Future ISBN: 978-1-53618-806-6
Editors: Joav Merrick et al.

Chapter 11

CROSS-SECTIONAL STUDY TO IDENTIFY RISK FACTORS FOR IMPAIRED EARLY CHILDHOOD DEVELOPMENT IN RURAL INDIA

Nandita Chattopadhyay, MBBS, DCH, DNB (Ped), FNNF, FAIMER Fellow, PG DiplDevNeurol*
Department of Paediatrics, IQ City Medical College, Durgapur, India

ABSTRACT

Healthy development in the early years provides building blocks for educational achievement, emotional and moral development. Enabling young children to achieve their full developmental potential is a requisite for sustainable development. Early childhood development (ECD) is affected by multiple adverse biological and socio-economic factors, exposure to which is commonly met with among the under-privileged. This study aims to assess the social and medical adversities faced by young children in the under-privileged rural community in India. A random sample survey was conducted in 523 households with children aged 0-6 years, in Eastern India, to identify the prevalent risk factors

* Corresponding Author's Email: chattnan@gmail.com.

deterrent to optimum brain development. Adversities like poor living conditions, lack of stimulatory home environment, learning opportunities and responsive parental care were identified. As a cumulative effect of these factors children were failing to achieve their developmental potential. Maternal education was the single most significant factor having an impact on these adversities and hence on ECD. Conclusion: Adequate education and empowerment of primary care-givers, especially mothers, can help to improve ECD.

INTRODUCTION

Early childhood is the foundation of future life. Healthy development in the first few years of life provides building blocks for educational achievement as well as emotional stability and morality. This leads to better economic productivity of the individual in adulthood and they grow up into responsible citizens, together building strong communities. It has been shown that an increased adult income in the new generation can break the intergenerational cycle of poverty and raise the human capital (1). In Jamaica children who were part of the early childhood home-visiting trials have now been followed into adulthood, showing sustained positive impact in terms of increased employment and earnings(2). Thus, to quote UNICEF, 'Early childhood development is the key to a full and productive life for a child and to the progress of a nation.'

All this will fail to be achieved if we do not focus on early childhood development in time. A study from the economic point of view shows that the cost of inaction today predicts a loss of 26% adult income/year (3).According to the World Health Organization, enabling young children to achieve their full developmental potential is a human right and a critical requisite for sustainable development. Evidence in the Lancet series 2017 (1, 4) called "Advancing early childhood development: From science to scale" served as a call to action globally.

Childhood development is key to achieving multiple sustainable development goals (SDG) including poverty reduction, nutrition, good health and wellbeing, school readiness and violence reduction (5-6). Governments and concerned stakeholders across the globe, today, are committed towards achieving the SDGs and global bodies like UNICEF, the World Bank and the World Health Organization have prioritized early childhood development in their agendas.

Early childhood development (ECD) is influenced by multiple biological and socio-economic factors. The socio-economic detrimental factors include violence at home, neglect, abuse, lack of opportunity for play and cognitive stimulation, and parental ill-health (7-8). Exposure to multiple such adversities is commonly met with among the under-privileged community in low- and middle-income countries (9-10). It is estimated that 250 million children (43%) less than five years of age in low and middle-income countries are at risk of suboptimal development (1).

Optimal child development starts before conception and is dependent on adequate nutrition for both, mother and child, protection from threats, provision of learning opportunities, and caregiver-interactions that are stimulating, responsive and emotionally supportive. This whole environment around a child has been conceptualized in the World Health Organization's "Nurturing care framework for early childhood development" (11-12), which was presented at the World Health Assembly in May 2018 to provide a roadmap for action.

Nurturing care consists of five inter-related components: health, nutrition, safety and security, early learning and responsive care. Children need all five domains of nurturing care to meet their developmental potential. The focus is on the first thousand days, the period from conception through the first two years of a child's life, because brain development progresses at a prolific rate during this period and neuroplasticity is at its peak (13).

Effective delivery of these five components will depend on an in-depth analysis of the socio-economic and cultural status of a community, so as to customize the deliverables for maximum impact. Many of the identified biological and socio-economic risk factors prevail among the under-privileged community in India, with a cumulative effect on ECD. Hence, before addressing the issue of ECD in rural India, we felt it prudent to assess the social and medical adversities faced by growing children, 0-6 years, in the under-privileged rural community.

In this study we undertook a random sample survey in a marginalized rural community in Eastern India, to identify the prominent risk factors prevalent in the area which may be deterrent to optimum early childhood development.

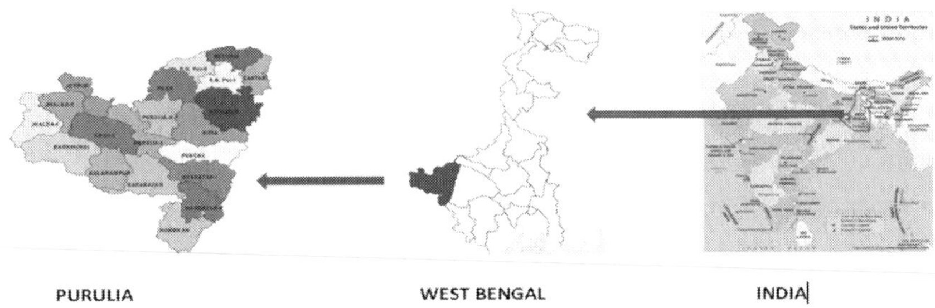

Figure 1.

OUR STUDY

Area of Study: Para Block in Purulia district of West Bengal was selected for the study. Para Block is divided into 10 Gram Panchayets (GP) or village counties, with total 119 inhabited villages and 28,462 households. We randomly selected 50+ households with children aged 0-6 years from each of these ten GPs (see figure 1). The study population was 523 families with children between 0-6 year age and the period January-March, 2019. The study is based on data collected from a door-to-door survey through a questionnaire based survey of randomly selected households. Attention was paid to include near equal representation from each of the 10 GPs. The questionnaire was designed by our expert team in line with the UNICEF MICS questionnaire, which included both closed and open-ended questions. Information was collected on the following:

- Details of the child's family: parents, other family members and siblings.
- Parents' occupation, education level, time spent with child.
- Details of home environment.

- Details of the child's exposure to early interventions at home and at ICDS centers.
- Scope for psychomotor stimulation at home.
- Attitude of care-givers towards child rearing and parenting skills.
- Child health and nutrition status.
- Child developmental status.

Special focus was laid on socio-cultural and socio-economic adversities which may affect child development. The collected data was checked for accuracy and consistency through vigilant scrutiny and then entered into a database. The data was analyzed using Microsoft EXCEL software. In tandem with the list of adversities used for an adversity score in the study conducted in Hariyana, India by Bhopal et al. (14) we focused on the following adversities:

- *Socioeconomic*: Mother's age, education and occupation, father's occupation (family income was not taken into account because all the families fell in the same income group, hence not a variable).
- *The child*: gender bias, born prematurely, high risk newborn/NICU graduate, inadequate care (child left alone or with a child under 10 years), parental awareness.
- *Home environment*: Home safety, stimulating environment, care-giver's involvement with child, parenting and discipline, harsh punishment.

FINDINGS

The study group comprised of 523 children from 0-6 years, with a mean age of 2.65 years. The male female distribution was 268:255, showing a male preponderance. Looking at the demographic profile, we found the following data:

1. Family structure was mostly joint family (412 out of 523).
2. Average number of family members was 9.5. 14 families had 20 or more members; highest family size recorded was with 50 members!
3. Number of siblings: 121 children had no siblings, 354 had 1-2 sibs while 3 or more sibs were seen in 48 families. Maximum number of siblings recorded was 11 (seen in two families).
4. Father's occupation in most families was either farming or as manual worker in brick kilns.
5. Mothers reported to be mostly housewives (470/523). Only 42 mentioned they worked in the fields, assisting in farming while 11 were involved in small businesses.
6. Age of mother: None were below 18 years and only 15 were between 18 and 20 years. 50 mothers were between 30-34 years while 25 were 35 years or more in age.
7. Maternal education: 112 mothers were illiterate, 203 had primary education, 158 had completed high school while 49 were graduates/post-graduates.

Home environment

253 families out of 523 lived in mud huts while 270 lived in brick houses. 76 (14.5%) families lived in a single room while 258(49.3%) had two rooms and 189 (36.1%) had three rooms. Average number of members in one room accommodations was 6.6 and maximum number of occupants noted was 19, indicating over-crowding. The rooms were mostly congested with poor ventilation. Natural light was adequate in 108 (20.6%), 291(55.6%) had moderate natural light indoors and in 124(23.8%) houses there was no or minimal natural light.

Stimulatory home environment

Locally available resources for early stimulations at home for infants and toddlers were available in most houses, though they were inadequately utilized to stimulate a baby or toddler. The things we looked for included simple toys, swing/hammock, wall-hanging pictures and calendars, mirrors, clocks and colorful linen. Based on availability of the seven common articles mentioned above, stimulatory environment was categorized as: Poor: 0-2 out of 7; moderate: 3-4 out of 7 and good:5-7 objects. Accordingly, 13% fell in the poor category, 19.2% in moderate and 67.4% were classified as good.

Home safety

Hazardous factors identified in the home environment which affect child safety include high cots, easy access to stove, fire, sharp objects, plastic bags, ponds, roads, inadequate fencing, tobacco, pesticides, hay stacks found around the house.Some Hazardous factors were identified in 78.7% households. Home safety was again classified as follows: 1-3 factors present: level 1 (mildly unsafe), 3-5 factors are present: level 2 (moderately unsafe) and 6-8 factors are present: level 3 (highly unsafe) (see Table 1).

Table 1. Safety level

Level of unsafe exposure	No. of children exposed (%)
Mild (level 1)	268 (51)
Moderate (level 2)	177 (34)
High (level 3)	78 (15)
Total	523

Parenting

99% mothers (housewife or working mothers), gave time to their children other than the feeding times, but mothers did not engage in interactive play or entertaining activities. Story-telling or reading books were not a common practice. Only 16.3% of mothers used paper, pencil and colors with children to encourage them to scribble or draw. Children played outdoors with other children, but a parent playing with them was not a common practice.67 (12.8%) children were reported to be left alone at home for more than an hour once or more in the last week, whereas they were reported to have been left with an older sibling in 145 (27.7%) homes. Fathers' involvement in childcare was common. Only 89 families reported that fathers were not spending time with the children. Peer mixing was commonly present. Only 25 families reported that their child did not get any peer time.

Parenting and child discipline

Permissive parenting with total lack of discipline was noted in 152 families (29%). Moderate punishment like slapping 218 (41.6%), yelling 323 (61.7%) was widely prevalent. Harsh punishment was regularly practiced in five families while 27 parents (5%) believed that physical punishment is necessary to raise a child. Only 62 children (12%) were exposed to positive parenting, where verbal abuse or physical assault was not being used to discipline the children. Their mistakes were being explained and told to rectify; things were not snatched away without explanations.

Pre-school attendance (ICDS centers)

68% children attend the government run free early education and pre-school centers(ICDS) regularly, but mostly because of the food they get there and not for the pre-school education services available (see Table 2).

Infants and toddlers were less frequently taken to the centre. The major focus was on 3-6 year olds. Mothers often did not accompany their children to the centers. Younger children were sent with the older siblings mostly to collect the food. Hence mothers were mostly unaware of the early Intervention and pre-school education facilities available at the ICDS. This points to poor utilization of available resources. Parents working in brick kilns relocate to the kiln site for months at a stretch, with the kids. During these prolonged periods of absence the children are forced to miss school.

Table 2. ICDS attendance according to age of child

Child Age	Goes to ICDS regularly (%)	Sometimes (%)	Never (%)	Total Children
0-2year	75(60)	26 (20.8)	24 (19.2)	125
>2 to 3 years	103(69)	31 (20.8)	15(10.1)	149
>3 to 4 years	109(71)	34(22.4)	9(5.9)	152
>4 years	68(70)	17(17.5)	12(12.4)	97
TOTAL (%)	355(68)	108(21)	60(11)	523

Child's health, nutrition, immunization and development

Number of children exclusively breast fed till six months: 433 out of 523 (82.7%). Number of children given complementary feeds from six months: 468 out of 523 (89.4%). Immunization of children was done regularly, though mostly depending on the health workers' reminders and immunization camps. Only 22% of mothers were aware of their child's next immunization dates (see Table 3). All families possess a health and immunization card, but awareness about its utility was inadequate. On enquiry, 315 out of 523 (60%) had no idea about the contents, while 175 mothers (33.4%) knew about immunization dates recorded in the card and only 34 mothers (6.4%) were aware of the health record and information maintained in the card.

Table 3. Maternal awareness about immunization dates

Criteria	No. of Mothers (%)
Mother looks for injection dates on health card	116(22.2)
Follow dates as advised by healthcare provider	259(49.5)
Follows health worker's advice and attends immunization dates	243(46.5)
Mother knows nothing about vaccines	21(4.0)

Developmental status

Developmental screening of all children through a simple questionnaire revealed that only 333 out of 523 (63.6%) children had fully attained the age-specific milestones. The rest 190 (36.4%) showed some delay, of whom 102 (19.5%) showed slight delay in the cognitive domain, possibly due to lack of proper stimulating environment and nurturing care. Out of them only three had associated gross motor delay, two had added fine motor delay and four had some speech delay. 60 children above 3 years showed an isolated delay in developing color perception, again possibly an effect of poor psychomotor stimulation. Six children had global developmental delay and 12 had cerebral palsy. Age wise distribution of developmental was also analyzed in Table 4. In most of the children lack of stimulation and opportunity had led to slight delay, most marked in 3-4 year olds. Color concept was strikingly absent in 3-4 year olds. Impact of these adverse factors on the child's development is shown in Table 5. Individually, none of the factors were found to have a significant influence on child development, except maternal education.

Table 4. Age-wise distribution of delay

	Total	Delay (%)	Remarks
<1yr	17	1 (5.8)	GM + FM
1-2	96	20 (20.8%)	Mostly GM, 3 CP/GDD
2-3	149	11 (7.3%)	Cog4 + Sp2 + GM4 + FM1 + GDD1
3-4	147	103 (70%)	Cog 60 + Color concept42 + Sp1 + GDD1
4-5	114	50 (43.8%)	Cog31 + Color concept 17 + Sp1 + GDD2

Legend: GM gross motor, FM fine motor, CP cerebral palsy, GDD global developmental delay, Cog cognitive, Sp speech.

Table 5. Impact of adversities on brain development

		no delay	delayed	p value
Siblings	3 or more	30	18	0.87
	<3	305	170	
Family size	7 or more	208	114	0.77
	<7	127	74	
Crowding	>5/room	14	15	0.48
	upto5/room	27	20	
Natural light	Poor	74	50	0.28
	adequate	261	138	
Home Safety	unsafe	265	147	0.82
	safe	70	41	
ICDS attendance	nil/irregular	109	58	0.84
	Regular	229	127	
Maternal Education	up to primary	184	132	0.0008
	High school and above	151	56	

Maternal education

Maternal education was seen to influence many of the parameters discussed above. So this factor was analyzed separately. The mothers' educational levels ranged from illiterate to post-graduates. Educational level of younger mothers was higher than the older mothers. Factors like family size, stimulating home environment, better child development, and awareness about health card were significantly affected by maternal education, while more deep-rooted circumstantial problems like environmental hazards remained unaffected (see Table 6 and Figure 2). Better educated mothers reported higher rate of illness in their children in the last one month than mothers with less education. Reporting of illness was also higher in families with less number of children (see Figure 3).

Table 6. Effect of maternal educational level on child rearing practices and awareness

Mother's education	Up to primary education: n = 315	High school-Graduate: n = 207	p-value	Remarks
No. of mothers having 3 or more children	129	22	<0.0001	Highly Significant
No. of households having poor stimulating environment for children	57	9	<0.0001	Highly Significant
Reads books to child	55	134	<0.0001	Highly Significant
Drawing/using pen & paper with child	65	75	<0.0001	Highly Significant
No. of houses having Hazardous environment for children	243	169	0.89	No significant difference
Knowledge of Immunization dates	78	97	<0.0001	Highly Significant
Knowledge about child development from Health card	17	17	0.2	No significance
Child attaining developmental potential	183	150	0.0008	Highly significant

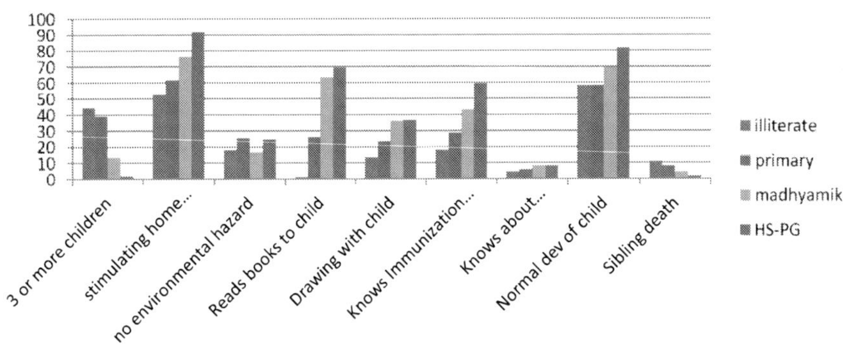

Figure 2. Effect on maternal education on socio-cultural factors and child rearing practices.

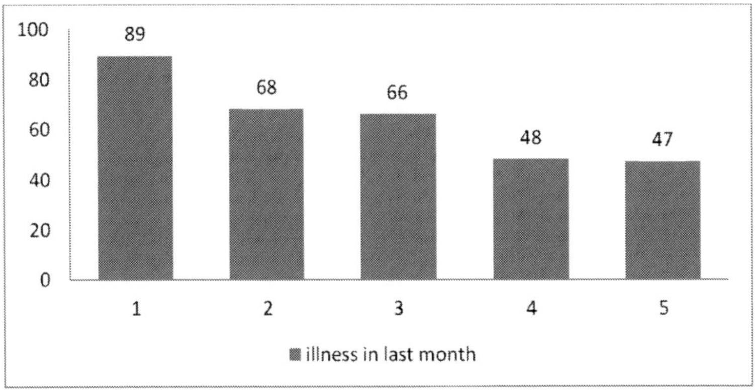

Figure 3. Child's illness in last month according to number of children.

Discussion

The community we surveyed was a marginalized rural community in West Bengal, India. The residents mostly lived in joint families. 90% of the families had up to three children; but in the rest 10% large numbers were noted with a maximum of 11 children in one nuclear family. The largest joint family had 50 members. Poverty was a common factor for all and the source of family income was farming, manual labor in farms and brick kilns and some cottage industry of which most common was binding of tobacco rolls (bidi).

89% of mothers declared to be housewives, though the figures may not be accurate, as many rural women had an inhibition to admit that they work for a living. Evidence of home-based production of tobacco rolls (bidi) was seen in most houses and womenfolk and older children were seen to be engaged in the activity. Handling tobacco leaves with bare hands and inhaling the tobacco laden air was a health hazard in itself.

Home safety was at stake in 78.6% houses. Parental occupation, lack of space and hygiene and social customs mostly led to these hazardous elements. Many of these factors, like tobacco dust in the air or husks, are difficult to eliminate as they are linked to deep-rooted socio-economic factors. The home environment was unhealthy with small, poorly ventilated and ill-lit rooms. Crowding was evident with an average occupancy of 6.6 per room. All this is detrimental to a child's well-being. Much of the poor environment can be improved by simple, low-cost measures, but that requires an awareness and motivation that is lacking among care-givers.

Early childhood development demands a home environment promoting psychomotor stimulation. Locally available resources for a young child's psychomotor stimulation, like wall-hanging pictures, mirrors, simple toys were available in most houses but their utilization for stimulating a child's early development was missing, again due to lack of awareness among care-givers. Most mothers spent adequate time with their children and were eager to help them, but they lacked the knowledge and skills to provide psychomotor stimulation. Interactive play, story-telling, reading books and encouragement to scribble and draw were markedly absent. This also was not because of non-availability but due to lack of awareness. Parents and care-givers did not focus on the child's developmental milestones unless they were grossly delayed. They had no notion on how to stimulate a child's development age-wise.

Coming to discipline, harsh punishments were rare, but proper positive parenting skills were also rarely practiced. Permissive parenting is commonly practiced and child rearing practices are not a major focus area.

Pre-school education and nutritional supplementation facilities are well available in the community through government run centers under the Integrated Child Development Scheme, but the facilities are under-utilized due to a communication gap between parents and providers.

So, to sum up, the adversities identified were poverty, poor housing, ill sanitation, over-crowding, health hazards at home, non-stimulating home environment, lack of parental awareness and poor parenting skills and poor utilization of available ECE resources like the ICDS centers. The severity of many of these factors was directly related to maternal education. These adversities showed a definite decline in families with educated mothers.

Our observations are comparable to a randomized controlled trial conducted in 2018 in Hariyana, India (14). This study was conducted in over 120 villages of rural India, where 1,273 children were assessed at 12 and 18 months of age for adversities in the first year of life. The association of adversities with growth and development in different domains was assessed. Consistent and strongly negative relationships were reported between all measures of childhood adversity. According to the study, most children faced one or more adversity and nearly 50% faced four or more, which impeded a child's well-being. Developmental assessment revealed up to 8 point fall in the cognitive and 11point fall in the language scale on BSID III. The authors inferred that these children were at risk of continuing suboptimal development through childhood (1). Another study by Agarwal et al. (15, 16) also reported associations between socio-economic status, family size and the home-inventory with developmental scores in 1–3 year olds in India.

We also came across studies from Bangladesh where Hamadani et al. (17) focused on socioeconomic status and home stimulation as measures of adversity and demonstrated an association with the mental developmental index. Other studies from Guatemala (18) and Ecuador (19) described a linear relationship between cumulative psychosocial risk and cognition development (10), while a Sri Lankan study demonstrated impaired development in children with increasing number of traumatic events (20).

With this socio-cultural background of adversities we tried to assess the developmental status of the children through a simple questionnaire. 36.4% of children showed some delay, of which 19.5% showed delay in the cognitive domain, possibly due to lack of proper stimulating environment and nurturing care. 60 children (11.4%) above 3 years of age showed an isolated delay in developing color perception, again possibly an effect of poor psychomotor stimulation. The slight cognitive delay we had noticed was most marked in 3-4 year olds. Color concept, which was strikingly absent among 3-4 year olds, was not so evident in 5 year olds, suggesting that these children were learning to identify colors around 5 years of age, in contrast, to children with good psychosocial stimulation, who invariably develop a color concept by 3.5 years of age.

Looking at the impact of the identified adverse factors on the child's development, surprisingly, we found that individually none of the factors had a significant influence on child development. This suggests that it is a cumulative effect of multiple factors that play a toll on brain development. The only single determinant that significantly affected the child's development was maternal education.

A gradual decreasing trend in family size and increasing trend in providing stimulating environment at home is noted with improved maternal education. Health hazards at home are almost equally present in all the groups, indicating that the social factors creating the hazards are not influenced by mothers' education. Often it is the family occupation that leads to health hazards. Maternal education improved the understanding and utilization of the health card, but even the well-educated mothers were not adequately conversant with the card. The child's developmental status was definitely better in case of educated mothers and sibling death reports were also much lower.

Surprisingly, better educated mothers reported higher rate of illness in their children in the last one month than mothers with less education. This could be due to lack of awareness of minor illnesses among the latter. The higher educated mothers showed more concern over minor illnesses which were overlooked by the former group. This finding corroborated with the fact that reporting of illness was higher in families with less number of children, the reason, probably was the same as above. Minor illnesses are not being reported or taken heed of in families with greater number of children and poorly educated mothers. A comparison showed that improved maternal education showed a positive trend in responsive care-giving and better early education for children.

To reach their full potential, children need the five inter-related and indivisible components of nurturing care (21), such as good health, adequate nutrition, safety and security, responsive care giving and opportunities for learning. In the first years of life, parents, intimate family members and caregivers are the closest to the young child and thus the best providers of nurturing care. So it is of utmost importance to address the parents and front-line workers and generate awareness about the five elements of nurturing care and a clear knowledge about what each component intends to deliver.

In the Indian scenario, healthcare and nutrition is addressed at every level and parents are reaping the benefits for their children through various Government schemes and programs in vogue. Issues regarding safety and security, responsive care giving and opportunities for learning are less attended to.

Security and safety (21) refers to safe and secure environments for children and their families, which includes protection from physical dangers, emotional stress, protection from physical punishment, abuse, and neglect, environmental risks like air pollution and access to food and potable water, availability of safe play area.

Opportunities for early learning (21) refers to any opportunity for the baby, toddler or child to interact with a person, place, or object in their environment. Every interaction (positive or negative, or absence of an interaction) contributes to the child's brain development and lays the foundation for later learning. The following measures are advocated to augment early learning:

- Using daily routines to talk to, play, and interact with baby/toddler/child.
- Telling stories.
- Exploring books together and reading to the baby/toddler/child.
- Smiling, imitating/copying, and simple games (e.g., peek a boo).

Responsive care giving (21) refers to the ability of the parent/caregiver to notice, understand, and respond to their child's signals in a timely and appropriate manner. Responsive caregivers are better able to support the other four components. Responsive care giving encompasses:

- Eye contact with baby, smile, cuddle, praise.
- Notice the child's cues and respond appropriately (sensitivity and responsiveness) – for example signs of hunger, satiety, illness, emotional distress, interest to play, pleasure.
- Try to identify and use everyday moments to communicate and play with their child.

- Develop safe and mutually rewarding relationships with their child so that they eventually enjoy being together.

To bring the nurturing care framework into action, the parents, especially the mother needs to be sensitized to all the above parameters. Only then can we rise above the adversities affecting early childhood development.

In order to improve early childhood development, WHO has endorsed the Nurturing Care Framework and has recently come up with the following recommendations (22):

- *Recommendation 1*: All infants and children should receive responsive care during the first three years of life; parents and other caregivers should be supported to provide responsive care.
- *Recommendation 2*: All infants and children should have early learning activities with their parents and other caregivers during the first 3 years of life; parents and other caregivers should be supported to engage in early learning with their infants and children.
- *Recommendation 3*: Support for responsive care and early learning should be integrated with interventions for optimal nutrition of infants and young children.
- *Recommendation 4*: Psychosocial interventions to support maternal mental health should be integrated into early childhood health and development services.

It is evident that emphasis lies on sensitization and empowerment of parents and primary care-givers to provide nurturing care, as they form the immediate environment of the child. Integration of services and delivery through a common portal is also important. It is only by educating primary care-givers, specially mothers and field level workers on child health and development that we can bring about an abatement of the socio-economic adversities, thereby augmenting early childhood development

CONCLUSION

Socio-economic and cultural adverse factors like poor health and hygiene, poor living conditions, lack of stimulatory home environment, learning opportunities and responsive parental care are prevalent among the under-privileged rural community in India, which hinder optimum development in young children. Most of these factors are strongly influenced by maternal education. Hence, these detrimental factors are likely to be overcome by adequate education and empowerment of primary care-givers, especially mothers, at the grass-root level. Our recommendations:

- Focus closely on improving security and safety, responsive care giving and opportunities for early learning
- Target parents and care-givers, especially mothers, for awareness generation and empowerment through duly trained field level workers
- Encourage peer interaction among mothers through mothers' meetings etc
- Involve community leaders in the program for better local participation. Inclusion of religious leaders may help in spreading the message of ECD
- Focus on education of girls, for better educated mothers in the coming days. Maternal education and empowerment is the single most effective factor in enhancing ECD.

ACKNOWLEDGMENTS

Ms Swati Basu, MSc (Stat) for data management and statistical analysis. Field staff of UDBHAAS Child Development Centre, NANRITAM for field work. Nanritam rural development campus, Para Block, District Purulia, West Bengal, India for logistic support. This study was funded by our organization, Nanritam. The author declares that they have no conflict of interest. Informed consent was obtained from each individual participant involved in this study. This study was conducted in accordance with the 1964 Declaration of Helsinki and its subsequent amendments. No animal was involved in this study.

REFERENCES

[1] Black MM, Walker SP, Fernald LCH, Andersen CT,DiGirolamo AM, Lu C,et al. Early childhood development coming of age: science through the life course. Lancet 2017;389(10064):77–90.

[2] Gertler P, Heckman J, Pinto R,Zanolini A, Vermeersch C,Walker S,et al. Labor market returns to an early childhood stimulation intervention in Jamaica. Science 2014;344(6187):998–1001.

[3] Advancing early childhood development: From science to scale. Executive summary, Lancet 2016 Oct:6-7. URL: https://www.thelancet.com/pb-assets/Lancet/stories/series/ecd/Lancet_ECD_Executive_Summary.pdf.

[4] Lu C, Black MM, Richter LM. Risk of poor development in young children in low-income and middle-income countries: an estimation and analysis at the global, regional and country level. Lancet Glob Health 2016;4(12):e916–22.

[5] Daelmans B, Darmstadt GL, Lombardi J,Dua T, Bhutta ZA, Richter LM, et al. Early childhood development: the foundation of sustainable development. Lancet 2017;389(10064):9–11.

[6] Sustainable Development Goals. URL: https://www.undp.org/content/undp/en/home/sustainable-development-goals.html.

[7] Cronholm PF, Forke CM, Wade R, Bair-Merritt MH, DavisM,Harkins-Schwarz M, et al. Adverse Childhood Experiences: Expanding the Concept of Adversity. Am J Prev Med 2015;49(3):354–61.

[8] Walker SP, Wachs TD, Gardner JM, Lozoff B, Wasserman GA, Pollitt E, et al. Child development: risk factors for adverse outcomes in developing countries. Lancet 2007;369: 145–157.

[9] Walker SP, Wachs TD, Grantham-McGregor S, Black MM, Nelson CA, Huffman SL, et al. Inequality in early childhood: risk and protective factors for early child development. Lancet 2011;378:1325–38.

[10] Wachs TD, Rahman A. The nature and impact of risk and protective influences on children's development in low-income countries. In:Britto PR, Engle PL, Super CM, eds. Handbook of early childhood development research and its impact on global policy. Oxford: Oxford University Press, 2013:85-122.

[11] Black MM, Trude ACB. Conceptualizations of child development benefit from inclusion of the nurturing care framework.J Nutr 2019;149(8):1307-8.

[12] Britto PR, Lye SJ, Proulx K, Yousafzai AK,Matthews SG,VaivadaT, et al. Nurturing care: Promoting early childhood development. Lancet 2017;389: 91–102.

[13] Shonkoff JP, Phillips DA, eds. From neurons to neighborhoods: The science of early childhood development. Washington, DC: National Academies Press, 2000.

[14] Bhopal S, Roy R, VermaD, KumarD, Avan B, Khan B,et al. Impact of adversity on early childhood growth & development in rural India: Findings from the early life stress sub-study of the SPRING cluster randomised controlled trial (SPRING-ELS). PLoS One 2019;14(1):e0209122.

[15] Agarwal DK, Awasthy A, Upadhyay SK, Singh P, Kumar J, Agarwal KN. Growth, behavior, development and intelligence in rural children between 1–3 years of life. Indian Pediatr 1992;29:467–80.

[16] Cox A, Walker S. The HOME Inventory.Brighton:Pavillion Publishing, 2001.

[17] Hamadani JD, Tofail F, Huda SN, Alam DS,RidoutDA,Attanasio O,et al. Cognitive deficit and poverty in the first 5 years of childhood in Bangladesh. Pediatrics 2014;134(4):e1001–8.

[18] Gorman KS, Pollitt E. Does schooling buffer the effects of early risk? Child Dev 1996;67(2):314–26.

[19] Paxson C, Schady N. Cognitive development among young children in Ecuador: The roles of wealth, health, and parenting. J Hum Resour 2007;42: 49–84.

[20] Catani C, Gewirtz AH, Wieling E, Schauer E, Elbert T, Neuner F. Tsunami, war, and cumulative risk in the lives of Sri Lankan schoolchildren. Child Dev 2010;81:1176–91.

[21] Five components of nurturing care: Nurturing care for early childhood development.URL: https://apps.who.int/iris/bitstream/handle/10665/272603/9789241514064-eng.pdf.

[22] Improving early childhood development: WHO guidelines URL: file:///F:/ECD%20material/WHO/9789240002098-eng.pdf.

SECTION TWO: ACKNOWLEDGEMENTS

In: Building Children and Youth for the Future ISBN: 978-1-53618-806-6
Editors: Joav Merrick et al.

Chapter 12

About the Editors

Joav Merrick, MD, MMedSci, DMSc, born and educated in Denmark is professor of pediatrics, Division of Pediatrics, Hadassah Hebrew University Medical Center, Mt Scopus Campus, Jerusalem, Israel and Kentucky Children's Hospital, University of Kentucky, Lexington, Kentucky United States and professor of public health at the Center for Healthy Development, School of Public Health, Georgia State University, Atlanta, United States, the former medical director of the Health Services, Division for Intellectual and Developmental Disabilities, Ministry of Social Affairs and Social Services, Jerusalem, the founder and director of the National Institute of Child Health and Human Development in Israel. Numerous publications in the field of pediatrics, child health and human development, rehabilitation, intellectual disability, disability, health, welfare, abuse, advocacy, quality of life and prevention. Received the Peter Sabroe Child Award for outstanding work on behalf of Danish Children in 1985 and the International LEGO-Prize ("The Children's Nobel Prize") for an extraordinary contribution towards improvement in child welfare and well-being in 1987. In 2017 appointed a Kentucky Colonel by the Commonwealth of Kentucky, the highest honor the governor can bestow to a person. Email: jmerrick@zahav.net.il

Ariel Tenenbaum, MD is the director of the Center for Children with Chronic Diseases at the Hadassah-Hebrew University Medical Center at the Mount Scopus Campus, Jerusalem, Israel. He graduated the Hadassah-Hebrew University Medical School and after pediatric residency at the Department of Pediatrics at Mount Scopus Campus, he continued his work at the hospital as a senior pediatric consultant and teacher of medical students. In 2004 he was appointed the head of the new Israeli Down syndrome program in the hospital. In 2005 he started the pre-adoption clinic together with Professor Isaiah D. Wexler. In 2012 he opened the Hadassah Intellectual and Developmental Disability Multidisciplinary Evaluation Center in collaboration with the Ministry of Social Affairs. He co-founded the Disability Studies Center at the Hebrew University, where he teaches students from humanities and social studies. He was recently appointed as a child development consultant. In 2019 he was elected to the Israeli Pediatric Association Committee and serves as its scientific secretary. His main research topics are disabilities, adoption, chronic diseases and general pediatrics. He has published numerous book chapters, edited several books, and published dozens of scientific articles in international journals. Email: tene@hadassah.org.il

Hatim A Omar, MD, FAAP, retired as Professor of Pediatrics, and Obstetrics and Gynecology at the University of Kentucky in Lexington until July 20, 2020 and served as founder and chief of the Division of Adolescent Medicine and Young Parent Program from November 1998 until December 2018. Dr Omar obtained his medical training at the Medical Academy, Sofia, Bulgaria, completed a residency in Obstetrics and Gynecology from Second United City Hospital, Sofia, Bulgaria and Pediatrics from West Virginia University, Morgantown, West Virginia and received postgraduate training in Adolescent Medicine at West Virginia University and Physiology at New York Medical College in Valhalla, New York. D. Omar is board certified in the areas of Pediatrics and Adolescent Medicine. He is the founder and Chairman of the Stop Youth Suicide Campaign. He served as a member of the Executive committee of the Section on Adolescent Health of the American Academy of Pediatrics and the Board of directors of the North American Society for Pediatric and Adolescent Gynecology. He has published extensively in all areas of care for adolescents in various peerreviewed scientific journals, books and many media outlets. He is on the editorial Board of the Journal of Pediatric and Adolescent Gynecology, International Journal of Adolescent Medicine and Health, Child Health and Human Development and four other peer reviewed journals. Dr Omar has served as an ambassador for wellbeing of adolescents world wide and is highly regarded for his tireless volunteer work on behalf of adolescents. Dr Omar is the recipient of: Founders of Adolescent Health Award: Community Leadership from the American Academy of Pediatrics: Section on Adolescent Health 2007; Special Achievement Award for bringing awareness to adolescent depression and suicide, American Academy of Pediatrics 2007; The Don Cantley Community Service award, Kentucky Pediatric Society 2007; SAAMY (Sexual Assault Awareness Month Award) for services to sexual abuse victims, presented by KY Association of Sexual Assault Programs 2007; Ohio Valley Society for Adolescent Medicine Award for dedication to adolescent health (for the Stop Youth Suicide Campaign) 2006; Commonwealth of Kentucky Governor's Award for Community Service and Volunteerism 2000; The William Lions Award, UK; Chairman's Research Award, Chairman's Teaching Award and the Miracle Maker Award in different years. He was recently appointed Kentucky Colonel, the highest civilian honor in the state of Kentucky. Email: 1958baladna@gmail.com

In: Building Children and Youth for the Future ISBN: 978-1-53618-806-6
Editors: Joav Merrick et al.

Chapter 13

About the National Institute of Child Health and Human Development in Israel

The National Institute of Child Health and Human Development (NICHD) in Israel was established in 1998 as a virtual institute under the auspices of the Medical Director, Ministry of Social Affairs and Social Services in order to function as the research arm for the Office of the Medical Director. In 1998 the National Council for Child Health and Pediatrics, Ministry of Health and in 1999 the Director General and Deputy Director General of the Ministry of Health endorsed the establishment of the NICHD.

Mission

The mission of a National Institute for Child Health and Human Development in Israel is to provide an academic focal point for the scholarly interdisciplinary study of child life, health, public health, welfare, disability, rehabilitation, intellectual disability and related aspects of human development. This mission includes research, teaching, clinical work, information and public service activities in the field of child health and human development.

Service and academic activities

Over the years many activities became focused in the south of Israel due to collaboration with various professionals at the Faculty of Health Sciences (FOHS) at the Ben Gurion University of the Negev (BGU). Since 2000 an affiliation with the Zusman Child Development Center at the Pediatric Division of Soroka University Medical Center has resulted in collaboration around the establishment of the Down Syndrome Clinic at that center. In 2002 a full course on "Disability" was established at the Recanati School for Allied Professions in the Community, FOHS, BGU and in 2005 collaboration was started with the Primary Care Unit of the faculty and disability became part of the master of public health course on "Children and society". In the academic year 2005-2006 a one semester course on "Aging with disability" was started as part of the master of science program in gerontology in our collaboration with the Center for Multidisciplinary Research in Aging. In 2010 collaborations with the Division of Pediatrics, Hadassah Hebrew University Medical Center, Jerusalem, Israel around the National Down Syndrome Center and teaching students and residents about intellectual and developmental disabilities as part of their training at this campus.

Research activities

The affiliated staff have over the years published work from projects and research activities in this national and international collaboration. In the year 2000 the International Journal of Adolescent Medicine and Health and in 2005 the International Journal on Disability and Human Development of De Gruyter Publishing House (Berlin and New York) were affiliated with the National Institute of Child Health and Human Development. From

2008 also the International Journal of Child Health and Human Development (Nova Science, New York), the International Journal of Child and Adolescent Health (Nova Science) and the Journal of Pain Management (Nova Science) affiliated and from 2009 the International Public Health Journal (Nova Science) and Journal of Alternative Medicine Research (Nova Science). All peer-reviewed international journals.

National collaborations

Nationally the NICHD works in collaboration with the Faculty of Health Sciences, Ben Gurion University of the Negev; Department of Physical Therapy, Sackler School of Medicine, Tel Aviv University; Autism Center, Assaf HaRofeh Medical Center; National Rett and PKU Centers at Chaim Sheba Medical Center, Tel HaShomer; Department of Physiotherapy, Haifa University; Department of Education, Bar Ilan University, Ramat Gan, Faculty of Social Sciences and Health Sciences; College of Judea and Samaria in Ariel and in 2011 affiliation with Center for Pediatric Chronic Diseases and National Center for Down Syndrome, Department of Pediatrics, Hadassah Hebrew University Medical Center, Mount Scopus Campus, Jerusalem.

International collaborations

Internationally with the Department of Disability and Human Development, College of Applied Health Sciences, University of Illinois at Chicago; Strong Center for Developmental Disabilities, Golisano Children's Hospital at Strong, University of Rochester School of Medicine and Dentistry, New York; Centre on Intellectual Disabilities, University of Albany, New York; Centre for Chronic Disease Prevention and Control, Health Canada, Ottawa; Chandler Medical Center and Children's Hospital, Kentucky Children's Hospital, Section of Adolescent Medicine, University of Kentucky, Lexington; Chronic Disease Prevention and Control Research

Center, Baylor College of Medicine, Houston, Texas; Division of Neuroscience, Department of Psychiatry, Columbia University, New York; Institute for the Study of Disadvantage and Disability, Atlanta; Center for Autism and Related Disorders, Department Psychiatry, Children's Hospital Boston, Boston; Department of Pediatric and Adolescent Medicine, Western Michigan University Homer Stryker MD School of Medicine, Kalamazoo, Michigan, United States; Department of Paediatrics, Child Health and Adolescent Medicine, Children's Hospital at Westmead, Westmead, Australia; International Centre for the Study of Occupational and Mental Health, Düsseldorf, Germany; Centre for Advanced Studies in Nursing, Department of General Practice and Primary Care, University of Aberdeen, Aberdeen, United Kingdom; Quality of Life Research Center, Copenhagen, Denmark; Nordic School of Public Health, Gottenburg, Sweden, Scandinavian Institute of Quality of Working Life, Oslo, Norway; The Department of Applied Social Sciences (APSS) of The Hong Kong Polytechnic University Hong Kong.

Targets

Our focus is on research, international collaborations, clinical work, teaching and policy in health, disability and human development and to establish the NICHD as a permanent institute in Israel in order to conduct model research.

Contact

Professor Joav Merrick, MD, MMedSci, DMSc
National Institute of Child Health and Human Development,
Jerusalem, Israel.
Email: jmerrick@zahav.net.il

In: Building Children and Youth for the Future ISBN: 978-1-53618-806-6
Editors: Joav Merrick et al.

Chapter 14

About the Center for Children with Chronic Diseases and Down Syndrome Center Jerusalem, Israel, Department of Pediatrics, Mt Scopus Campus, Hadassah Hebrew University Medical Center, Jerusalem, Israel

Chronic illnesses are common among children. These conditions last longer than a year and require continuous medical care and special needs. It is estimated that 10-20% of children in developed countries have one or more chronic condition. Advances in medicine and technology lead to an increase in the survival rate and longevity of children with chronic diseases and special needs. The severity of different chronic illnesses is variable, but there are many similarities. The child with a chronic illness faces physical, social, and emotional challenges. Therefore, medical care is not sufficient without rehabilitative service and emotional care for the child and his family.

Chronic illnesses are time and energy consuming. These children go through treatments, procedures and many healthcare visits. At home they often continue treatments as well, e.g., physiotherapy, breathing support machines and medications. This lifestyle may have detrimental effect on the child's social and emotional well-being, and similarly affect his parents and siblings.

Center for Children with Chronic Diseases

The aim of the Center for Children with Chronic Diseases at the Hadassah-Hebrew University Medical Center at the Mount Scopus Campus, Jerusalem, is to enhance medical care, comfort and well-being of patients and their families in the hospital and beyond. The center provides integrated and comprehensive care for these patients. This includes extensive support services and helping their families cope with the burden of care.

Numerous pediatric specialty programs and medical divisions have been established in the center to care for specific chronic conditions; among them are cystic fibrosis, Down syndrome, diabetes mellitus, familial dysautonomia, neuromuscular diseases, rheumatic diseases, feeding disorders and metabolic diseases. All these programs include evaluation and support from common services in the center: Nursing, nutrition, psycho-social care, speech therapy, physiotherapy and more.

The center works as a "one stop shop" for these children; As many services as possible, under one roof, on the same visit. Centralizing the care enables parents to come to one location to receive care. The physicians and nurses coordinate the care of the children thereby alleviating some of the burden of care off the families.

Children who are included in the programs of the center usually need returning visits to various medical specialists, consultations by multidisciplinary health professionals and performing diagnostic tests e.g., blood work, x-rays and respiratory functions. Some children may need hospitalization or palliative care. The center can concentrate all diagnostic and follow-up testing, medical surveillance and treatment in the hands of an experienced staff who knows the child and his unique situation.

The center is situated close to the entrance of the hospital and the families can access it without going through the main hospital building. In the center there are ten rooms for consultations. In addition, there are dedicated rooms for tests, e.g., respiratory functions, blood tests, sweat test and more. There is a large space with eight beds for continuous treatments, for example intravenous immunoglobulins and biological medications. In this space several unique tests are performed as well, for example growth hormone test and allergy challenge tests. There is also a special room for procedures, in which children can go through painful treatments with appropriate anesthetics and surveillance.

A special classroom in the center is operated by the ministry of education. In the classroom, children can continue their studies or play and interact with other children, in arts and crafts and many other programs.

The center is surrounded by a large healing garden that is partially maintained by the children themselves.

Conclusion

In conclusion, we believe that the "all inclusive" model of a center for children with chronic conditions is beneficial for the children and their families in terms of health and quality of life, and that this model is currently the best service for them.

Contact

Ariel Tenenbaum, MD, Isaiah D Wexler, MD, PhD
Center for Children with Chronic Diseases, Department of Pediatrics,
Mt Scopus Campus, Hadassah Hebrew University Medical Center,
Jerusalem, Israel
Email: TENE@hadassah.org.il

In: Building Children and Youth for the Future ISBN: 978-1-53618-806-6
Editors: Joav Merrick et al.

Chapter 15

THE ANNUAL "STOP YOUTH SUICIDE" CONFERENCE, LEXINGTON, KENTUCKY, UNITED STATES

In October 2000, the Stop Youth Suicide Campaign was launched (see stopyouthuicide.com) with the following goals in mind:

- Increase awareness about youth suicide in the community, schools and homes
- Advocacy to create state wide suicide prevention
- Develop a grassroot program to actually reduce teen suicide completions and attempts

As part of the effort, a state conference was held in February 2001. Although we never had actual funding, we still wanted parents, teens and school personnel to be able to attend at little or no cost. I recruited caring experts from around the world to help by being speakers with no financial compensation. The initial conference was a great success, which led me to organize another one in November 2001 and to make it an annual event since.

The conference is held in the month of November each year in Lexington, Kentucky, generally the 1st week unless there is a conflict with other events in the city.

A total of 18 conferences have been held since then and every topic related to teen health is usually addressed. We want to educate people about teen development, and the factors leading to risky behavior including suicide. Throughout the years, we have always been filled to capacity and the evaluations are always very positive.

Moving forward, we will continue to update participants on the newest knowledge about teens and engage the community as a whole in overall prevention of risk behavior.

Contact

Hatim Omar, MD, FAAP
Founder of the Stop Youth Suicide Campaign
Lexington, Kentucky, United States
Email: 1958baladna@gmail.com
Website: stopyouthsuicide.com

SECTION THREE: INDEX

INDEX

C

D

E

F

G

H

I

Q

R

S